Acknowledgements

To my child. Everything I do, I have done it for you. I love you more than words can say. I hope you get the opportunity to make this world a better place.

To Dr. MB. Many, many thanks. Your words still echo in my head and heart.

Disclaimer

This book is not intended to treat, diagnose, cure, prevent disease, nor is it offering medical advice of any kind. The research and opinions presented in this book is the work of the author. Please consult your physician or medical provider regarding any treatment or medical needs that you may have.

This book is not to be taken in place of legal advice or legal consideration. The author is not a lawyer and is not licensed to practice law. Legal opinions are strictly that of the author.

I wrote this book as a health care provider and as a person who is absolutely appalled at the American health care system today. The American public is being sold out (and in some cases, fraudulently so) so doctors, schools, Congress, and health care facilities can make a few extra dollars, and this is not something that sits well with me. I did not join the medical profession to force medical treatment upon my patients. I did not become a nurse to get rich or to harm people. Autonomy, personally and professionally, has always been important to me. I am also aware that some of what I write here may ruffle a few feathers.

Health care workers need to know that their employer is mandating that they have an ineffective and forced medical treatment so that they do not lose funding. College students have the right to know that their professors are receiving kickbacks from pharmaceutical companies in return for not fully providing information on medication and medical procedures; or for providing them with false information due to conflict of interest or ethics violations. The American public deserves to know and understand that their representatives in Congress are being bought and paid for by a pharmaceutical company that wants to keep its product on the shelves even though they are killing people. Patients have the right to know that they can be sold out for a dollar. Furthermore, patients, and health care workers alike need to know that there is rampant fraud in research (all aspects), and that any research should be heavily scrutinized and taken with a grain of salt, and any conflicts of interest should be noted.

I recently came across a book written by an American doctor who examines his own greed and how easy it was to become corrupt, but also how easy it was to get caught. His book, if interested, is *Confessions of an American Doctor.* This was heartbreaking and enlightening to read, particularly as I was in the middle of completing my research for this book.

I hope that if nothing else a dialogue can open, and discussions can be had regarding financial incentive, privacy, and personal autonomy in health care. I hope that patients don't have to choose between their insulin for the month and paying the light bill. And above all else, I hope that people finally start demanding answers that have long since been covered up, and that eyes are opened to how the human body here in the US is being exchanged for profit.

Dr. Amelia M. Kenyon
DNP, MSN, RN

Book Contents

Chapter 1

<u>Government Health Agencies</u>

"Those who do not learn from history are doomed to repeat

it."

George Santayana

Government health agencies in the United States have been known to make much ado about nothing, have participated in horrific human experiments, and have hidden a lot of their misdeeds from the public. Many of these assaults on humanity have been done for the purposes of obtaining funding. From the CDC, to the NIH, to the FDA, at one time or another, human subjects have been traded for a few dollars. And in some cases, for many millions of dollars.

Many Americans are (somewhat) aware of the Tuskegee Syphilis Experiments done in the African American Community in from the 1930's to the early 1960's. However, are you aware of the forced sterilization programs across the US that happened from the early 1900's to the 1970's? Prisoners in the US have made fine specimens for experimental medical projects. Have you heard about the studies done on the mentally ill throughout the 1900s? The University of Michigan performed flu experiments spraying live specimens in mental institutions in the 40's. We can only begin to guess what type of experiments have been done to our American soldiers and are very likely continuing to occur. Though I understand that Wikipedia is not considered a reliable source of information for research purposes, feel free to look at the page on human experimentation in the United States and then investigate a little bit further. I believe that many of the references in Wikipedia can lead to solid and informational resources. The amount of unethical treatment of persons in the US is astounding and frightening: https://en.wikipedia.org/wiki/Unethical_human_experimentation_in_the_United_States

One of the best sources of information that truly examines human experimentation, ethics, and the potential financial impact is "The Immortal Life of Henrietta Lacks" by Rebecca Skloot (2010). In her book on Ms. Lacks, Rebecca Skloot explores many unethical tactics that were used to obtain the cancer cells of Henrietta Lacks (HeLa) and distribute them to various research centers all over the world. Mrs. Lacks and her entire family were duped during the extraction of cells and the attempt to collect more data on her children and husband. Her family, by the way, received no funding, no compensation, and little acknowledgment to the advancements that have been made regarding Mrs. Lacks' cell usage. Scientists have made millions of dollars selling these cells and receiving funding for the research being completed using these cells. It is worth noting, however, that millions of dollars have also been lost due to the HeLa cells tainting many levels of research and studies, which has generated more money being given and spent.

Mrs. Lacks was not the only person that this happened to. A gentleman named John Moore from California also had his cells taken and used experimentally. Mr. Moore sued the physician who took his cells claiming he had the rights to his own cells and body parts. Scarily enough, the California Supreme Court ultimately ruled against him stating discarded blood/cells/tissues are not the personal property of the person from whom they were removed (Campbell, 2006). I personally believe that Mr. Moore might have won his case had he not been trying to profit from it financially, and fought for medical privacy, such as was done in Roe vs. Wade. On the other hand, should a physician be able to take *your* discarded/unattached/removed body tissue and then profit from a cell line creation? What about ethics violations? This is walking a very tight and slippery rope.

Lately on social media sites such as Facebook and Twitter, genetic companies have been advertising swab studies for you to receive information about your ancestry or medical history. While many people are excited about this, they fail to read the fine print where it says that these companies can basically do what they please with your test results. While these are not government agencies per se, they can certainly report your private medical information and your genetic information to government agencies, per their terms of service. Here is one example from the company GeneSight: ("Assurex Health," 2017)

How else can we use or share your health information? We are allowed or required to share your information in other ways – usually in ways that contribute to the public good, such as public health and research. We have to meet many conditions in the law before we can share your information for these purposes. For more information see: www.hhs.gov/ocr/privacy/hipaa/understanding/consumers/index.html.

Help with public health and safety issues	We can share health information about you for certain situations such as: Preventing disease; Helping with product recalls; Reporting adverse reactions to medications; Reporting suspected abuse, neglect, or domestic violence; Preventing or reducing a serious threat to anyone's health or safety
Do research	We can use or share your information for health research.
Comply with the law	We will share information about you if state or federal laws require it, including with the Department of Health and Human Services if it wants to see that we're complying with federal privacy law.
Respond to organ and tissue donation requests	We can share health information about you with organ procurement organizations.
Work with a medical examiner or funeral director	We can share health information with a coroner, medical examiner, or funeral director when an individual dies.
Address workers' compensation, law enforcement, and other government requests	We can use or share health information about you: • For workers' compensation claims • For law enforcement purposes or with a law enforcement official • With health oversight agencies for activities authorized by law • For special government functions such as military, national security, and presidential protective services

And the organization 23AndMe states that they will release your information for research, unless you specifically tell them otherwise ("DNA Testing," n.d.). (The consent forms are signed when you agree to initial testing.)

8. 23andMe Privacy Statement and Disclosure of Information

In order to use the Services, you must first acknowledge and agree to the Privacy Statement. You may not use the Services if you do not accept the Privacy Statement. You can acknowledge and agree to the Privacy Statement by (1) clicking to accept or agree to the Privacy Statement, where this option is made available to you by 23andMe for any Service; or by (2) actually using the Services.

You acknowledge and agree that 23andMe has the right to monitor any use of its systems by its personnel at any time and maintain copies documenting such monitoring. Our Privacy Statement sets forth the only expectations of privacy any individual should have in terms of usage of the 23andMe Services, website or other systems. If you have given consent for your Genetic Information and Self-Reported Information to be used in 23andMe Research as described in the applicable Consent Document, we may include your information in the Aggregated Genetic Information and Self-Reported Information we disclose to third parties for the purpose of publication in a peer-reviewed scientific journal. 23andMe may also include your information in Aggregated Genetic and Self-Reported Information disclosed to third-party non-profit and/or commercial research partners who will not publish that information in a peer-reviewed scientific journal. 23andMe Research may be sponsored by, conducted on behalf of, or in collaboration with third parties, such as non-profit foundations, academic institutions or pharmaceutical companies. 23andMe Research may study a specific group or population, identify potential areas or targets for therapeutics development, conduct or support the development of drugs, diagnostics or devices to diagnose, predict or treat medical or other health conditions, work with public, private and/or non-profit entities on genetic research initiatives, or otherwise create, commercialize, and apply this new knowledge to improve health care. 23andMe will never release your individual-level Genetic Information and/or Self-Reported Information to any third party without asking for and receiving your explicit consent to do so, unless required by law.

As a consumer and as a medical professional, I would be very cautious about sending any DNA samples to any of these organizations. The fact remains, is that we don't really know what they are doing with the private medical information that they collect, and I would personally be very hesitant to submit to any genetic testing in this manner. You can do as you please, but buyer beware if you decide to participate in something such as this. Don't think for one minute that you truly have privacy if you are participating with one of these genetic testing organizations.

In 2015, the Centers for Disease Control (CDC) took it upon themselves to create a "crisis" out of an Ebola outbreak that was currently going on in Africa at the time. They brought patients over to the United States, to treat them here, versus sending a specialized team overseas. They allowed nurses to treat patients without proper treatment protocols or proper training. Registered nurses working in the US obtained the virus due to improper training and protocols in place at their places of employment. (And of course, these nurses were blamed for contracting the disease, as if it was their fault.) The women who contracted the disease suffered terribly. For months, all we heard about was the potential Ebola crisis here in the United States. Then, suddenly, we hear nothing. (Newsflash: Ebola is still occurring in various parts of Africa.) It has been suggested that this "crisis" was created so the CDC could request more funding ("Ebola," 2017).

The CDC has a history of abusing the funds that the American taxpayer provides them. In 1999, an investigation determined that the CDC misspent $23 million dollars that was earmarked for a chronic fatigue syndrome study, and then lied about it to Congress (Strauss, 1999).

In 1976, the swine flu that hit the United States was hyped and advertised as "the worst crisis of all time" and encouraged everyone to receive an experimental vaccine. The swine flu itself killed just one person, hospitalized 13, yet there were hundreds of injuries and deaths from the experimental vaccine that was rushed into production. There were many calls for accurate reporting of information, as the government nearly created a panic regarding the swine flu. It turned out to be much ado about nothing (Roan, 2009).

During the AIDS epidemic in the 80's, the US government and the CDC was hardly an example of a reliable source. They suspected as early as the first quarter of 1982 that the disease was caused by a virus, and that it was very likely sexually transmitted because of the rate that it was spreading among sexually active gay men across the country. They also knew of the virus' long latency period before eruption into full-blown AIDS as well. Furthermore, the CDC also allowed blood banks to continue to use blood donated by those who had the virus well after it was determined that this could turn up in the bloodstream. The CDC did little to quell the panic that you could obtain AIDS by touching or kissing someone, and they became the go-to source of (very bad) information during this time. Some have even suggested that the CDC was looking for a new disease at the time because they were afraid that funding was going to run out. They were also afraid to "offend" a minority group, as AIDS in the US was primarily occurring in young, homosexual men. They felt that by suggesting that they use protection, or abstain from sex, would be telling them what they could do with their own bodies. Rather than saving lives, they took the PC approach to the virus, and this allowed it to spread even further and longer than it probably should have (Shilts, 1988).

In his book, "AIDS and the Doctors of Death," Dr. Alan Cantwell suggests that AIDS was a man-made disease introduced into the gay communities in the late 70's via the Hepatitis B experiments that were operated by Dr. Wolf Szmuness. Dr. Cantwell's very well researched book suggests that during the 1970's, cancer researchers wanted to determine that cancer could be caused by a virus. (Many of these researchers used the HELA cells stolen from Henrietta Lacks and sold on the medical market.) Dr. Cantwell explores the fact that many viruses were contaminated, cross-contaminated, and combined in many various ways (Cantwell, 1988). Cantwell further suggests that serious ethics violations have occurred by many government agencies in the last several decades, and that it continues today.

The United States military is also no stranger to experimentation when it comes to enlisted soldiers. The 1950's included experiments on soldiers such as Project Bluebird and MKUltra. The latter of which partnered with the United States Central Intelligence Agency (CIA) to perform tests on both civilians and military personnel. (Some conspiracy investigators allege that MKUltra projects continue to this day.)

In the 1960s, the military experimented with nerve gas on soldiers aboard ships during the Project Shipboard Hazard and Defense projects that were established from 1963-1969. These tests and experiments were designed to see how the US military could withstand chemical attacks. However, soldiers were not informed of the tests, nor were they given informed consent about participation.

Every year for the last twenty years, the CDC and the mainstream media claim that we are in the "worst flu season of all time;" however, the actual numbers to back this claim don't add up. For the 2014-2015 flu season, there were 691,952 specimens tested for influenza. Of these, only 125,462 specimens tested positive for influenza. These specimens come from doctor's offices, urgent cares, hospitals, med centers, and other lab testing sites. This is a far cry from the "millions of Americans" who get the flu each year. This also means that out of those who report with "flu-like symptoms" to their doctor, hospital, urgent care, or med center, there is about an 18% chance of them having influenza.

On top of this it was confirmed that 141 children died of influenza that same year. This means that during the 2014-2015 flu season, a child had an extremely low chance of dying of influenza. How many adults died? That number is unobtainable for about three years. Why? Because the CDC lumps influenza and pneumonia together to create their number in the interim. Never mind that they are two totally separate and completely different illnesses. They do this to create the illusion that influenza is a far worse virus than it is. The CDC also mentions that most of the adult cases of influenza, also have a co-disorder such as heart disease, CHF, diabetes, COPD, and other lung diseases. They also admit that nearly 75% of the adult cases, are in those over the age of 65.

However, they do release the data about three years later. The report for 2014 was released in 2017, and the information is shown below:

Cause of death (based on ICD-10)	All ages	Under 1 year	1–4	5–14	15–24	25–34	35–44	45–54	55–64	65–74	75–84	85 and over	Age not stated
All other forms of heart disease ... (I25–I29,I34–I38,I42–I49,I51)	132,525	273	116	148	696	1,622	3,198	7,670	14,198	20,039	31,167	53,389	9
Essential hypertension and hypertensive renal disease .. (I10,I12,I15)	30,221	2	1	–	20	108	439	1,429	3,382	4,464	7,023	13,374	–
Cerebrovascular diseases ... (I60–I69)	133,103	93	33	99	177	679	1,716	5,040	11,707	18,003	36,333	57,292	4
Atherosclerosis ... (I70)	6,356	3	–	2	2	4	26	116	393	749	1,488	3,573	–
Other diseases of circulatory system ... (I71–I78)	19,199	14	3	7	47	170	414	1,007	2,341	3,846	5,272	6,077	1
Aortic aneurysm and dissection ... (I71)	9,863	–	1	2	32	114	302	659	1,348	2,048	2,744	2,612	1
Other diseases of arteries, arterioles and capillaries ... (I72–I78)	9,336	14	2	5	15	56	112	348	993	1,798	2,528	3,465	–
Other disorders of circulatory system ... (I80–I99)	4,548	15	1	5	49	136	354	603	815	791	823	955	1
Influenza and pneumonia ... (J09–J18)	55,227	166	109	98	199	549	1,125	2,731	5,390	7,861	13,193	23,792	4
Influenza ... (J09–J11)	4,605	30	39	53	54	165	350	583	900	618	715	1,098	–
Pneumonia ... (J12–J18)	50,622	156	70	45	145	384	775	2,148	4,490	7,243	12,478	22,684	4
Other acute lower respiratory infections ... (J20–J22,U04)	289	38	18	4	4	6	11	16	22	20	38	112	–
Acute bronchitis and bronchiolitis ... (J20–J21)	232	36	16	3	4	5	10	15	20	14	24	85	–
Other and unspecified acute lower respiratory infections .. (J22,U04)	57	2	2	1	–	1	1	1	2	6	14	27	–
Chronic lower respiratory diseases ... (J40–J47)	147,101	19	53	139	178	367	754	4,402	16,492	35,617	47,758	41,318	4
Bronchitis, chronic and unspecified ... (J40–J42)	563	14	19	2	5	10	14	21	55	96	117	211	–
Emphysema ... (J43)	7,455	2	1	1	1	6	39	327	1,039	1,944	2,412	1,683	–
Asthma ... (J45–J46)	3,651	2	29	130	161	283	357	577	586	435	441	650	–
Other chronic lower respiratory diseases ... (J44,J47)	135,432	1	4	6	11	68	344	3,477	14,812	33,143	44,788	38,774	4
Pneumoconioses and chemical effects ... (J60–J66,J68)	737	–	2	–	–	–	2	7	47	135	292	252	–
Pneumonitis due to solids and liquids ... (J69)	18,792	5	6	7	46	91	160	529	1,332	2,482	5,015	9,108	1
Other diseases of respiratory system ... (J00–J06,J30–J39,J67,J70–J98)	36,197	269	114	72	116	236	511	1,529	4,237	7,825	10,981	10,497	–
Peptic ulcer ... (K25–K28)	3,027	2	–	3	4	27	73	201	518	552	717	931	–

(Kochanek et al., 2016)

So how many people died of the actual influenza in 2014? 4,605.

In 2012, that number was around 1200. Keep in mind that this number does not drastically change from year to year. Out of a population of 380 million persons living in the United States, I'd say this makes the chances pretty good! You are more likely to be killed by a medical error, heart attack, or diabetes. In fact, you are probably more likely to die falling over your own two feet than you are by influenza. (Yes, this number is included in the report as well!)

> *Fall*—In 2014, 33,018 persons died as the result of falls, 16.5% of all injury deaths (Table 18). The age-adjusted death rate for falls increased 3.4%, from 8.8 in 2013 to 9.1 in 2014. The overwhelming majority of fall-related deaths (96.8%) were unintentional.

(Kochanek et al., 2016)

It should also be noted, that when the CDC provides information to the public, all the references supplied are from government funded, or CDC interested groups, parties, or studies. There are no independent studies offered to the public at all. You can see this for yourself first hand here:

https://www.cdc.gov/mmwr/volumes/65/wr/mm6537a5.htm?s_cid=mm6537a5_w

"The U.S. influenza surveillance system is a collaboration between CDC and federal, state, local, and territorial partners and uses nine data sources to collect influenza information, seven of which operate year-round. During May 22–September 10, 2016, laboratories participating in the U.S. World Health Organization (WHO) Collaborating Laboratories System (primarily public health laboratories) tested 5,365 specimens for influenza and 817 were positive for seasonal influenza viruses; 458 (56.1%) were influenza A viruses, and 359 (43.9%) were influenza B viruses. Influenza B viruses were reported more frequently than influenza A viruses during May–June. However, since the beginning of July, influenza A viruses were reported more frequently. Of the 448 influenza A viruses subtyped, 377 (84.2%) were influenza A (H3N2) viruses and 71 (15.8%) were influenza A (H1N1) pdm09 viruses. Lineage was determined for 249 influenza B viruses; 172 (69.1%) were B/Yamagata lineage and 77 (30.9%) were B/Victoria lineage. During the same period, laboratories participating in the National Respiratory and Enteric Virus Surveillance System (NREVSS) (primarily clinical laboratories) tested 110,230 specimens for influenza viruses; 2,126 (1.9%) were positive. Among the positive specimens, 763 (35.9%) were influenza A viruses and 1,363 (64.1%) were influenza B viruses. Influenza viruses were reported from Puerto Rico and 49 states in all 10 U.S. Department of Health and Human Services regions" (CDC Weekly MMR, 2017).

You also have organizations such as the AAFP "bragging" when a vaccine is 50% effective. (50% is a failing rate in any grading scale that I have seen or used.) (http://www.aafp.org/news/health-of-the-public/20170221fluvacceffect.html)

The CDC further states that "It is not possible to predict which influenza virus will predominate, how severe influenza-related disease activity will be, or how effective influenza vaccine will be during the 2016–17 season. However, since February 2016, CDC's laboratory-based studies of approximately 5,000 influenza viruses found that most circulating viruses do not have significant antigenic changes" (CDC MMR, 2017).

In 2014 the CDC confirmed that 17,911 persons were hospitalized with influenza between October 1, 2014- April 30th, 2015. (The final death tally for this will be available in 2018.) It is impossible for 30,000 people a year to die of influenza based on these numbers. The CDC, the media, and anyone else (including physicians and medical organizations) who give these numbers is lying to the American public. It must stop. Providing false information to the public, researchers, and medical staff does nothing but perpetuate fear and create concern where there is none.

The CDC does not have America's best interest at hearts. They appear to align many of their teachings and information with whatever the pharmaceutical companies want us to hear. On top of that, we also need to wonder if they aren't setting us up for a mutated influenza virus that will be deadly and will account for numerous patient deaths. We all took high school biology class. Viruses and bacteria mutate. They do this to survive. The vaccines are clearly not working. We have heard every year for the last few years that the viruses are mutating beyond the protective level for the flu vaccine, effectively rendering the vaccine ineffective. (Which it is anyway, as they admit to the "guesswork" that goes into the creation of the vaccine each year.)

In the last two years, the CDC has taken it upon themselves to create a panic over the Zika virus. Along with the CDC, the American media came together to raise the alarm, and it has appeared that there has been much ado about nothing. We heard news stories of nurses who were at risk, and nurses who contracted the disease, and then the blame game began. Nurses were not trained and ill-prepared to handle incoming cases obtained the disease and then were blamed for doing so (Askt, 2014). On top of the blame, the rumors spread like wildfire that every American was now at risk for the disease and we were all going to potentially die. Fortunately, it turned out to be much ado about nothing, but it was not without a large scare tactic from the government and the US media.

Ultimately nurse Nina Pham sued and settled with her employer after contracting the disease. Her name, likeness, etc. were spread throughout the media and social media without her consent or her awareness, and while she was desperately ill. She continues to suffer with side effects today (Emily, 2016).

It should go without saying that government agencies do not always have our best interests at heart. Being suspicious of a government entity does not make one a "conspiracy theorist" or a "nut-job," rather a consumer or citizen who is aware and wishes to remain aware of what is going on in his/her health and country.

Chapter 2

Congress, the Lobbyists, and the Political Buyout of Professional Organizations

"The American Republic will endure until the day Congress discovers that it can bribe the public with the public's money."

Alexis de Tocqueville

"...all members of Congress should be required wear NASCAR uniforms. You know, the kind with the patches? That way we'd know who is sponsoring each of them."

—Brad Thor, Full Black

It is no secret that many members of Congress are heavily influenced by pharmaceutical companies and their lobbyists. What does continue to be a secret is the exact financial level that this influence is ingrained into our lawmakers, business, and professional organizations. There are many out there, and this chapter will explore this in detail.

In looking at the financial disclosures of members of Congress, one must wonder how a Congress person making $174,000 a year is able to afford a multi-million-dollar home. Take Ms. Maxine Waters for instance. Maxine is a Congress woman from Los Angeles, CA. Maxine represents one of the poorest communities in California, yet she can afford a five-million-dollar home. She can apparently afford to pay her daughter a $750,000 per year salary to mail out her fliers and mailers each year. So, how DOES a Congress person from such a poor district afford such riches? Note that she also does not live in the district she keeps getting elected in either. (Silly me; I thought that was a requirement!)

Looking at Maxine's financial disclosure summary only adds more questions. She apparently has two other mortgages in the amounts of about $500,000 each as well. Her income is only listed; not her spouse's. After doing a quick calculation, there is no way someone with a $174,000 per year salary, even with excellent credit scores and a 0% interest rate, could afford these houses on this income. You may wonder why I am using this as an example. I do this because it has been shown time and time again that many members of Congress are heavily influenced and supported by pharmaceutical companies in the United States. Some disclose this information, but many do not.

Recently, Congresswoman Nancy Pelosi was called out about her financial conflicts of interest. While she lectured constituents on inordinate wealth, she refused to answer calls about her own financial inordinate wealth. Bizarrely, she went on a rant about being a "mother of five" and refused to answer any questions (Ernst, 2018). It is worth noting that both Pelosi and Waters are both senior citizens and are over the age of 75. Both women have served in Congress for many decades, and this has been their main "job" in life. To the best of my knowledge, there are no medical exams done in Congress to determine if someone is mentally or physically capable of doing the job that they are elected for. This sets for a poor precedent as to who is representing the American people.

Lobbyists, are ruining and running our country. Many millions of dollars are being exchanged to keep Americans and their health at the bottom of the barrel. Pharmaceutical companies have nearly endless pocketbooks and they are very happy to open those to people who have no qualms about being "purchased" to promote an agenda or a cause.

One of the best websites that monitors the influence that pharma, insurance, and medical companies have on our government officials is the Union of Concerned Scientists. Their website spells out in full detail what they look for, and the conflicts of interest that exist within our current government.

http://www.ucsusa.org/our-work/center-science-and-democracy/promoting-scientific-integrity/drug-companies-influence-FDA.html#.WcKI4meWypo

"Data compiled by the Center for Responsive Politics and commissioned by the Union of Concerned Scientists show that between 2009 and 2011, prescription drug, biotechnology and medical device companies spent more than $700 million lobbying Congress and the Obama administration.

That's a lot of money. By comparison, the insurance industry spent $480 million in the same period. Drug companies alone spent more than $487 million on lobbying during the three-year period; biotechnology and medical device companies spent $126 million and $86 million, respectively.

Over the same period, elected officials on a House subcommittee and a Senate committee with oversight over FDA received nearly $6.3 million in campaign contributions from these industries. Donations went to both Republicans and Democrats"

The website and organization, Open Secrets: Center for Responsive Politics shows the following graphics demonstrating where pharmaceutical companies have spent regarding lobbying and Congressional pressure in the last decade:

(https://www.opensecrets.org/industries/indus.php?ind=H04)

Top Contributors, 2017-2018

(Move your cursor over the chart to see dollar amounts.)

Contributor	Amount
Pfizer Inc	$638,053
De Shaw Research	$539,404
Amgen Inc	$456,823
Exoxemis Inc	$450,000
AmerisourceBergen Corp	$401,483
Eli Lilly & Co	$351,822
Express Scripts	$348,299
Abbvie Inc	$345,280
Johnson & Johnson	$313,699
Merck & Co	$311,466
Sanofi	$286,510
Starkey Hearing Technologies	$270,103
Health Foods of America	$252,800
Abbott Laboratories	$243,346

Top Lobbying Clients, 2017

Client/Parent	Total
Pharmaceutical Research & Manufacturers of America	$14,227,500
Amgen Inc	$6,620,000
Novartis AG	$5,879,510
Pfizer Inc	$5,690,000
Bayer AG	$4,970,000

This chart is particularly interesting because it shows a rather large spike in 2008- the same year that the Affordable Care Act was passed:

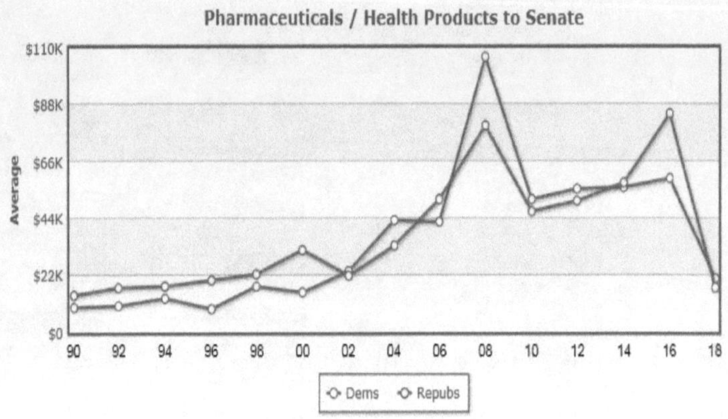

From the group United Republic, they demonstrate that lobbyists also encourage higher drug prices.

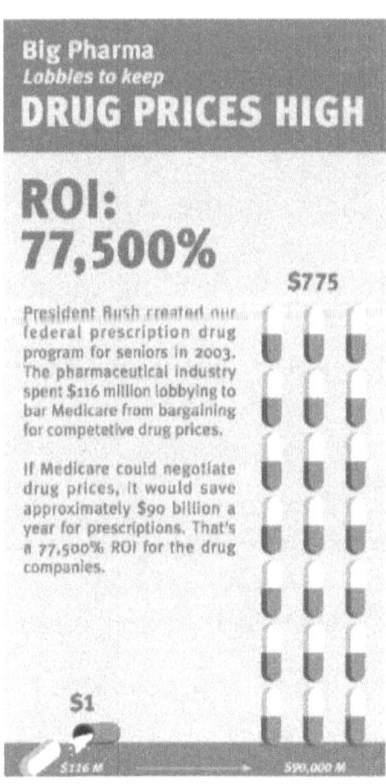

In 2016, the American Nurses Association made the decision to endorse a presidential candidate. This ultimately ended up backfiring when dozens of complaints hit their social media sites with many members pulling their memberships from the ANA over their candidate choice (ANA, 2016). It has become clear in recent years that the ANA and other professional medical associations have chosen to be mouthpieces for various causes and this is probably due to donations and funding coming from unethical and unscrupulous sources.

The ANA claims that the support came from their political action committee, but at any rate, it did not sit well with many members. Speaking of members, how many are there in the ANA? Well, that number is unknown. The ANA claims to be "the leading member-based organization for registered nurses in the USA" but they don't publish their membership numbers. This is suspicious. The website http://www.unionfacts.com lists the membership level at 172,107- a far cry from the 3.6 million that they claim to represent:

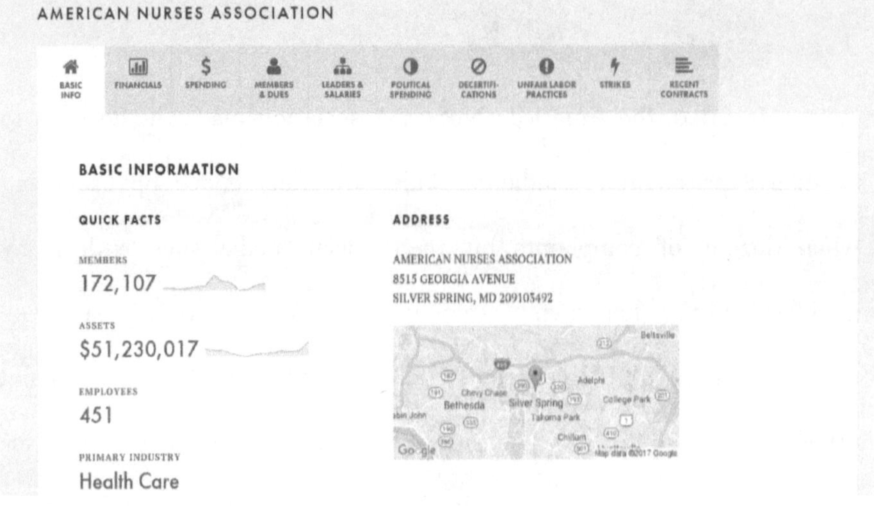

(Union Facts, n.d)

The ANA membership is not cheap either. You must click through about 10 screens before you can find the cost on their website. They want you to sign up for an account before they will show you the prices of their memberships. Dues are around $200 per year. If that is the case, then, they don't have nearly the 172,000 members that they claim. According to UnionFacts, they have 14,577,958 coming in from dues-membership fees. That number, divided by the $200 membership fee per person, comes to 72,889 members- about 100,000 less than reported to Union Facts.

INCOME

Dues	$14,577,958
Per Person Tax	$0
Investments	$21,854,270
Supplies	$0
Loan Repayment	$0
Interest	$0
Dividends	$0
Rents	$372,549
Fees and Fines	$0
Loans Obtained	$0
Other Receipts	$43,679,040
Affiliates	$8,035,652
Members	$51,564
Reinvestments	$5,195,360
All Others	$2,503,026

(Union Facts, n.d)

What does the money go for? Well $50 a year goes to their magazine publication that they send out. This is basically a mouthpiece for the ANA, and whatever pet topics they have been paid to support or promote that month. There is nothing with real substance in it. Members can get CEUs and access to journal articles, but the actual membership is really nothing more significant than a piece of paper.

The ANA claims to be an organization representing nurses, but they are legally classified as a labor union. This can be verified with the United States Department of Labor's website.

What is particularly concerning regarding the ANA is the fact that they publish the "Code of Ethics" for nurses. This "code of ethics" guides many schools of nursing, health care facilities, hospitals, and more. On top of their poor choice of support for a presidential candidate, they also do not have a good reputation as an employer. The reviews of the ANA on Glassdoor are quite damning, and more than a little frightening. https://www.glassdoor.com/Reviews/American-Nurses-Association-Reviews-E355881.htm

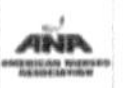

"Dread going to work..."

▼ Current Employee - Anonymous Employee

🔳 Doesn't Recommend   🔳 Negative Outlook   🔳 Disapproves of CEO

I have been working at American Nurses Association full-time (More than 3 years)

Pros

Location, benefits, hours, flexibility and work/life balance

Cons

Bullying allowed by management
Directors don't protect staff
Racial tension
Lack of diversity in senior management
Leadership does not live the values
Minorities held to different standards

Advice to Management

- Dismiss directors leading departments with high turnover...where there's smoke, there's fire
- Diversify your leadership...no minority leading a department in 2017 is glaring
-Hold directors accountable for living values

May 29, 2017   Helpful (12)

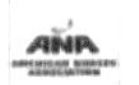

"Toxic environment of bullies"

▼ Former Employee - Anonymous Employee in Silver Spring, MD

🔳 Doesn't Recommend   🔳 Negative Outlook   🔳 Disapproves of CEO

I worked at American Nurses Association full-time (More than 10 years)

Pros

Lots of dedicated non management employees who genuinely care about nurses.

Cons

LOOK AT THE NUMBER OF REVIEWS WITH THUMBS UP THAT ARE NEGATIVE COMPARED TO POSITIVE REVIEWS FROM FORMER EMPLOYEES. It's a TERRIBLE place to work!

Ironic that a major issue ANA wants to help nurses address is workplace bullying when it is so egregious and rampant at their offices. It is very telling that during the time I was there, the entire HR department turned over three or four times. They even outsourced ...

Show More

Advice to Management

Fear, intimidation and bullying is not a way to inspire and get the best out of your employees.

Stop trying to implement yet another work group or survey, or study to address lack of communication and collaboration. Why would anyone want to stick there necks out to help others when there is a track record of people doing so and begin punished or

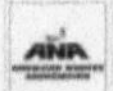

"Run, Don't Walk Away, From This Failing Organization..."

 Current Employee - Anonymous Employee in Silver Spring, MD

Doesn't Recommend   **Negative Outlook**   **Disapproves of CEO**

I have been working at American Nurses Association full-time (More than 3 years)

Pros

Benefits, Birthday Off, Recently Remodeled Office

Cons

Highly Incompetent Managers, Seldom Seen Executive Leadership, Silo Mentality Among departments, Uncreative & Unimaginative Vision, Spiteful and Trifling Employees

Advice to Management

You have your hands full in turning around this failing organization. You need managers who actually have management experience and stop hiring employees who are like everyone else.

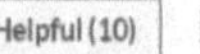

Helpful (10)

Feb 16, 2017   Helpful (10)

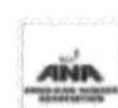

"Toxic Culture that plague organization still prevalent in long-time staff members"

  Current Employee - Anonymous Employee

Doesn't Recommend   **Negative Outlook**   **No opinion of CEO**

I have been working at American Nurses Association full-time (Less than a year)

Pros

location, salary, some benefits. efforts to change organization into a more positive, nurturing work environment. 3% auto raise every Feb.

Cons

Depending on which department you are in, bullying and intimidation persist despite cultural transformation push. unrealistic expectations of work and deadlines. staff does more than job description says. manipulative, cliquish, and petty behaviors run rampant. union environment. lack of engagement from senior-level management in employee conflicts. people expect you to know what you don't know about how the organization works. lack of accountability. more concerned about making a profit than the mission, but the organization is losing money.

Show Less

Advice to Management

fire the last of the folks who are part of the old culture.

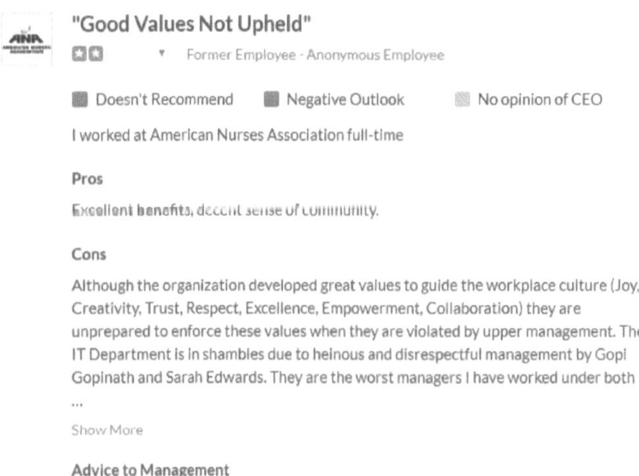

(Glassdoor, 2017 and 2018)

And these are just a few of the examples. Is this really the organization that we want representing nurses? Or that claim to be the best association for nurses to be associated with? An organization that clearly doesn't follow its own Code of Ethics? With the lack of transparency that they possess, and the fact that they are not willing to release true membership numbers, the political stances that they choose, and the fact that they appear to be bought out, the ANA should not be looked to as a model organization for nurses. Nurses need to step up and start questioning the ethics of this so-called nursing organization.

Towards the end of 2017, the CEO of the ANA stepped down. Marla J. Weston resigned as of January 1, 2018 ("ANA Resignation," 2017). It is interesting to note that poor reviews on Glassdoor and other websites of the organization have continued.

I chose to examine the ANA in this chapter for the very reasons listed above. There is far too much secrecy, favoritism, and lack of transparency within their organization to truly support professional nurses. They also do not offer much in exchange for their pricey membership. Some nurses consider it prestigious if they can state that they are a member, but ultimately, it doesn't mean or account for much.

No other country in the world has their health care system run by lobbyists, financial incentives, conflict of interest, or pharmaceutical companies. This must stop, and it must be reconciled.

To the best of my knowledge and research, I am unable to locate anything that requires the reporting of payments, payoffs, etc. by pharmaceutical companies to our Congressmen and women. Yes, they are required to submit financial disclosures, but the reality is, is that is not happening. I believe that some of the payoffs may be occurring in real estate transactions, off the record cash transactions, and even overseas to hide the financial influence that is occurring within our government. Congress is not going to create laws that may stop this influence, so it is up to the American people to investigate and report on any findings that they come across that shows any potential ethical conflicts.

Chapter 3

<u>**Hospitals Selling Employee's Bodies? Say It Isn't So!**</u>

"Truth telling and medicine don't go together except in

dire emergencies, if then."

Mario Puzo

Do you have mandatory flu vaccine policies in place at your hospital? Are you told that this is done in the name of "patient safety?" Did you also know that your employer receives a large chunk of money each year for proving that they have a large percentage of staff vaccinated against the flu? Don't be alarmed, most people don't know this either. And the hospitals will lie through their teeth before they will admit to this! I wrote another book that explores this in much more depth titled "Legal and Ethical Problems with Mandatory Vaccine Policies in the Workplace." It is also available for sale and explores many more resources or health care workers that I am only going to briefly touch upon on this chapter.

After World War 2, and the horrors of what happened under Nazi Germany were discovered, countries came together to form what is now known as the Nuremberg Codes. These codes discussed human experimentation and what was expected of studying human subjects. There are ten points in the code, and they first and foremost state:

"The voluntary consent of the human subject is absolutely essential. This means that the person involved should have legal capacity to give consent; should be so situated as to be able to exercise free power of choice, without the intervention of any element of force, fraud, deceit, duress, over-reaching, or other ulterior form of constraint or coercion; and should have sufficient knowledge and comprehension of the elements of the subject matter involved, as to enable him to make an understanding and enlightened decision. This latter element requires that, before the acceptance of an affirmative decision by the experimental subject, there should be made known to him the nature, duration, and purpose of the experiment; the method and means by which it is to be conducted; all inconveniences and hazards reasonably to be expected; and the effects upon his health or person, which may possibly come from his participation in the experiment" ("Nuremberg," 1949).

Informed consent means that patients are fully informed of the *risks* and the benefits of any medical procedure. Very few patients can say that they have truly given informed consent before they are given a vaccine. Many of the "informational sheets" that are handed out do not list vaccine ingredients, adverse effects, or what to do in the case of a reaction (https://www.cdc.gov/vaccines/hcp/vis/). Summarily, the reporting and the information on what to do for an adverse event is not given, and many nurses and health care workers themselves cannot describe what to do in the case of an adverse event. This is a devastating fact in the health care field and one that should be remedied and taught in all schools of medicine.

Since the passing of the Affordable Care Act (ACA), organizations that accept Medicare and Medicaid can participate in the Hospital Value-Based Purchasing (HVBP) program set forth by the ACA. In 2013, it was established that reimbursement rates under the ACA and the HVBP is tied in part to employee influenza vaccination rates ("Quality Reporting," 2011). A large percentage of health care systems, have created mandatory vaccination policies for employees in their organizations ("Payment Adjustments," n.d.). They have done this, so they do not lose out on a potential 2% bonus incentive that has come along with the HVBP program. Most of these organizations have little or no exemptions for medical, religious, or philosophical beliefs. Some organizations require employees wear a mask (if a refusal or exemption is given), which potentially violates employee privacy (Landro, 2013). Most employers have also not informed their employees that the vaccination policy is being tied into government reimbursement. The information regarding this from the government is difficult to locate. These mandatory policies are setting a potentially illegal and unethical precedent.

According to the Centers for Disease Control (CDC), the flu vaccine is estimated to be only about 60% effective in its best year ("Vaccine Effectiveness," 2015). However, the Cochrane Collaboration suggests the flu vaccine is only about 10% effective in any given year. Their recommendation is that no healthy adult be vaccinated against the influenza as it appears to not work and has little to no benefit (Jefferson et al., 2014). As we discussed earlier, deaths from influenza are extremely rare, and the true numbers of death are combined with pneumonia deaths per the CDC ("Estimating Death," 2015). More people die each year from heart disease, diabetes, hospital errors, and accidents ("Cause of Death," 2015). The last two years the CDC has admitted that the flu vaccine has not been effective and has offered little protection for those who have taken it ("Protection Reduced," 2015).

Every single year, news media reports that "the flu shot is the best way to reduce the risk of getting sick," yet the numbers regarding the effectiveness of the influenza vaccine don't support this statement. Health care workers are told that the best way to prevent illness and the spread of infection is hand washing, yet as discussed in chapter one, about half of health care workers don't wash their hands like they should.

The CDC's website estimates the effectiveness of a flu vaccine to be around 50-60% each year ("Vaccine Effectiveness," 2017). This estimate gives a person a 50/50 chance of being protected. However, when you look at effectiveness studies that the CDC provides on its website, you will notice that the actual effective rate is not anywhere near these numbers:

Influenza Season[†]	Reference	Study Site(s)	No. of Patients[‡]	Adjusted Overall VE (%)	95% CI
2004-05	Belongia 2009	WI	762	10	-36, 40
2005-06	Belongia 2009	WI	346	21	-52, 59
2006-07	Belongia 2009	WI	871	52	22, 70
2007-08	Belongia 2011	WI	1914	37	22, 49
2008-09	Unpublished	WI, MI, NY, TN	6713	41	30, 50
2009-10	Griffin 2011	WI, MI, NY, TN	6757	56	23, 75
2010-11	Treanor 2011	WI, MI, NY, TN	4757	60	53, 66
2011-12	Ohmit 2014	WI, MI, PA, TX, WA	4771	47	36, 56
2012-13	McLean 2014	WI, MI, PA, TX, WA	6452	49	43, 55
2013-14	Gagiani 2009	WI, MI, PA, TX, WA	5999	52	44, 59
2014-15	Zimmerman 2016	WI, MI, PA, TX, WA	9311	19	10, 27
2015-16*	ACIP presentation, Flannery [332 KB, 26 pages]	WI, MI, PA, TX, WA	7563	47*	39, 53*

*Estimate from Nov 2, 2015–April 15, 2016.

("Seasonal Effectiveness," 2016).

Viral and bacterial mutation are rarely if ever mentioned. The strains selected each year, per the CDC's admission, are guesses as to what may be floating about the next year. The World Health Organization (WHO) states, "characteristic of many RNA genome viruses, influenza virus undergoes high mutation rates and frequent genetic reassortment (combination and rearrangement of genetic material) leading to variability in HA and NA antigens. Minor changes in the protein structure in influenza A strains ("antigenic drift") occur frequently, enabling the virus to cause repetitive influenza outbreaks by evading immune recognition" (WHO, 2016).

A recent study released in 2017 states:

"The impression that unvaccinated HCWs place their patients at great influenza peril is exaggerated. Instead, the HCW-attributable risk and vaccine-preventable fraction both remain unknown and the NNV to achieve patient benefit still requires better understanding. Although current scientific data are inadequate to support the ethical implementation of enforced HCW influenza vaccination, they do not refute approaches to support voluntary vaccination or other more broadly protective practices, such as staying home or masking when acutely ill" (Serres et al., 2017).

The study by Serres et al. completed four randomized controlled trials in long-term care facilities to observe for their study. Their ultimate results stated, "more realistic recalibration based on actual patient data instead shows that at least 6000 to 32,000 hospital workers would need to be vaccinated before a single patient death could potentially be averted" (Serres et al., 2017). This study demonstrates that the idea that health care workers are "saving lives" by receiving a flu vaccine is simply a lie.

In 2014 the Cochrane Collaboration issued a study that ultimately concluded "Influenza vaccines have a very modest effect in reducing influenza symptoms and working days lost in the general population, including pregnant women" (Jefferson et al., 2014). The study looked at over 116 studies for the influenza vaccine before making their conclusion. This study along with the Serres study should be taken seriously when considering forcing influenza vaccines on employees. Both studies demonstrate that the flu vaccine is not effective in "protecting patients" and provides a modest coverage, if any at all.

The idea of patient autonomy supports a patient's right to refuse

medical treatment or procedure (Craigie, 2011). When a health care

worker is on the receiving end of a needle, he or she is no longer just an

employee but is now also a patient. In the same way that their patients

have the right to refuse medical treatment, the same principle should

ethically and legally apply to the health care worker as well. If a health

care worker is to become injured by the mandatory vaccine, he or she is

unable to sue the vaccine manufacturer ("FAQ," n.d.). The injured health

care worker could file a complaint with the Vaccine Injury Compensation

Program via the Vaccine Adverse Events Reporting System (VAERS).

There is no guarantee of compensation though, and it could take years to

reach a settlement. The legal burden may lie on that of the health care

system who mandated the vaccine for the health care worker to retain

employment with their organization. An employee injury due to

mandatory vaccination could prove very costly for that health care

system. Many health care organizations force their employees to sign

waivers stating that they will not hold the hospital responsible the case of

an injury.

Consider this scenario: a patient requests a new nurse/caregiver because that nurse is wearing a mask. This nurse has a legitimate medical reason for not receiving the influenza vaccine, yet as punitive punishment, they are made to wear a mask. Could the health care organization be held liable for this? Isn't this quite the same as a patient requesting a new caregiver because they don't want a caregiver of the opposite sex/age/race, etc.? Yes, it is. The employee's rights have been violated, their right to medical privacy has been put on display, and the employer is now set up to be sued.

Title VII of the Civil Rights Act of 1964 ("EEOC," n.d.) prohibits employer discrimination based on race, religion, color, sex, or national origin. Many health care professionals have legitimate religious concerns or beliefs regarding vaccines. Some may differ from their religion's official stance, but these are deeply held religious beliefs, which are protected by law (Grabenstein, 2013).

The Equal Employment Opportunity Commission (EEOC) has also weighed in on religious rights in the refusal of a mandatory vaccination. They support the right of a health care worker to refuse a mandatory vaccination based on a "sincerely-held" religious belief. The EEOC states that an employer who terminates an employee based on this refusal due to religious beliefs may be violating the law. If the employee sincerely believes that it is against their beliefs to have the injection, the burden lies with the employer to not discriminate. The EEOC also makes it clear to health care organizations that making employees jump through hurdles (i.e. Having a signed letter from clergy or a religious mission statement) is also a violation of the law ("EEOC Opinion," 2012). Many employees continue to be denied religious exemptions even after leaping through these hoops (Bruce, 2016). Thankfully, the EEOC is going after employers who are doing this and violating their employees' religious beliefs.

Upon learning that she is pregnant, an expectant woman is told to avoid caffeine, tobacco, alcohol, and common drugs like Tylenol or Ibuprofen. However, many employers are mandating that pregnant/nursing employees be forced into taking a flu vaccine, or face termination. Many employers are also breaking the law when it comes to these mandates.

The EEOC states that not accommodating a pregnant woman who wishes to refuse the vaccine, may put an employer in violation of the Pregnancy Discrimination Act (PDA) ("EEOC Opinion," 2012). This can cause the employer to be held liable for damages in the case of a pregnant employee suing or facing termination due to flu shot refusal.

In 2013, Goldman's research demonstrated that there was a significant risk of miscarriage for a pregnant woman following administration of the flu vaccine. Goldman stated, "The observed reporting bias was too low to explain the magnitude increase in fetal-demise reporting rates in the VAERS database relative to the reported annual trends. Thus, a synergistic fetal toxicity likely resulted from the administration of both the pandemic (A-H1N1) and seasonal influenza vaccines during the 2009/2010 season (Goldman, 2013)". Goldman goes even further to ascertain "The VAERS rates of 6.8 and 12.6 fetal-loss reports per million women vaccinated for those single-vaccine seasons may provide health care professionals with a sense that influenza vaccines administered during pregnancy are relatively safe, when these rates merely reflect the low level of case ascertainment associated with VAERS and thus, grossly underestimate the true rates encountered in the US population."

Further studies also suggest that even low doses of mercury administered in the first trimester can be harmful to a developing fetus. Brow and Austin (2012) summarized their study by stating: "Data demonstrated that Hg exposures, particularly during the first trimester of pregnancy, at well-established dose/weight ratios produced severe damage to humans including death. Considering research suggestive of a mercuric risk factor for childhood conditions such as tic disorders, cerebral palsy, and autism, it is essential that Hg advisories account for secondary prenatal human exposures." Though this writer discussed this in chapter four, a screen shot of the Fluzone vaccine is shown below:

1   **Table 6: Fluzone Quadrivalent Ingredients**

Ingredient	Quantity (per dose)	
	Fluzone Quadrivalent 0.25 mL Dose	Fluzone Quadrivalent 0.5 mL Dose
Active Substance: Split influenza virus, inactivated strains[a]:	30 mcg HA total	60 mcg HA total
A (H1N1)	7.5 mcg HA	15 mcg HA
A (H3N2)	7.5 mcg HA	15 mcg HA
B/(Victoria lineage)	7.5 mcg HA	15 mcg HA
B/(Yamagata lineage)	7.5 mcg HA	15 mcg HA
Other:		
Sodium phosphate-buffered isotonic sodium chloride solution	QS[b] to appropriate volume	QS[b] to appropriate volume
Formaldehyde	≤50 mcg	≤100 mcg
Octylphenol ethoxylate	≤125 mcg	≤250 mcg
Preservative		
Single-dose presentations	-	-
Multi-dose presentation (thimerosal)	12.5 mcg mercury	25 mcg mercury

2   [a]per United States Public Health Service (USPHS) requirement

("Fluzone," 2016)

Flu vaccine inserts state "safety and effectiveness have not been established in pregnant women or nursing mothers" ("Fluarix," 2015; "Fluzone," 2016; "Flucelvax," 2016). Furthermore, the vaccine insert goes on to state that "FLUARIX should be given to a pregnant woman only if clearly needed" ("Fluarix," 2015, p. 10).

HIGHLIGHTS OF PRESCRIBING INFORMATION
These highlights do not include all the information needed to use FLUARIX safely and effectively. See full prescribing information for FLUARIX.

FLUARIX (Influenza Vaccine)
Suspension for Intramuscular Injection
2015-2016 Formula
Initial U.S. Approval: 2005

---------------------------**INDICATIONS AND USAGE**--------------------
FLUARIX is a vaccine indicated for active immunization for the prevention of disease caused by influenza A subtype viruses and type B virus contained in the vaccine. FLUARIX is approved for use in persons 3 years of age and older. (1)

--------------------- **DOSAGE AND ADMINISTRATION** ----------------
For intramuscular injection only. (2)

Age	Vaccination Status	Dose and Schedule
Aged 3 through 8 years	Not previously vaccinated with influenza vaccine	Two doses (0.5-mL. each) at least 4 weeks apart (2.1)
	Vaccinated with influenza vaccine in a previous season	One or two doses[*] (0.5-mL. each) (2.1)
Aged 9 years and older	Not applicable	One 0.5-mL dose (2.1)

[*] One dose or two doses (0.5-mL. each) depending on vaccination history as per the annual Advisory Committee on Immunization Practices (ACIP) recommendation on prevention and control of influenza with vaccines. If two doses, administer each 0.5-mL. dose at least 4 weeks apart. (2.1)

------------------- **DOSAGE FORMS AND STRENGTHS** -------------
Suspension for injection supplied in 0.5-mL. single-dose prefilled syringes. (3)

------------------------------**CONTRAINDICATIONS**-----------------------
History of severe allergic reactions (e.g., anaphylaxis) to any component of the vaccine, including egg protein, or following a previous dose of any influenza vaccine. (4, 11)

-------------------- **WARNINGS AND PRECAUTIONS** ----------------
* If Guillain-Barré syndrome has occurred within 6 weeks of receipt of a prior influenza vaccine, the decision to give FLUARIX should be based on potential benefits and risks. (5.1)
* Syncope (fainting) can occur in association with administration of injectable vaccines, including FLUARIX. Procedures should be in place to avoid falling injury and to restore cerebral perfusion following syncope. (5.2)

-------------------------- **ADVERSE REACTIONS** -----------------------
* In adults, the most common ($\geq$10%) local and general adverse events were pain and redness at the injection site, muscle aches, fatigue, and headache. (6.1)
* In children aged 5 years through 17 years, the most common ($\geq$10%) local and general adverse events were similar to those in adults but also included swelling at the injection site. (6.1)
* In children aged 3 years through 4 years, the most common ($\geq$10%) local and general adverse events were pain, redness, and swelling at the injection site, irritability, loss of appetite, and drowsiness. (6.1)

To report SUSPECTED ADVERSE REACTIONS, contact GlaxoSmithKline at 1-888-825-5249 or VAERS at 1-800-822-7967 or www.vaers.hhs.gov.

-------------------- **USE IN SPECIFIC POPULATIONS** ----------------
* Safety and effectiveness of FLUARIX have not been established in pregnant women or nursing mothers. (8.1, 8.3)
* Register women who receive FLUARIX while pregnant in the pregnancy registry by calling 1-888-452-9622. (8.1)
* In a clinical trial of children younger than 3 years, antibody titers were lower after FLUARIX than after an active comparator. (8.4)
* Geriatric Use: Antibody responses were lower in geriatric subjects who received FLUARIX than in younger subjects. (8.5)

See 17 for PATIENT COUNSELING INFORMATION.

Revised: XX/201X

("Fluarix," 2015)

* In adults $\geq$65 years of age, the most common injection-site reaction was pain (>20%); the most common solicited systemic adverse events were headache, myalgia, and malaise (>10%). (6.1)

To report SUSPECTED ADVERSE REACTIONS, contact Sanofi Pasteur Inc., Discovery Drive, Swiftwater, PA 18370 at 1-800-822-2463 (1-800-VACCINE) or VAERS at 1-800-822-7967 or www.vaers.hhs.gov.

------------------------**USE IN SPECIFIC POPULATIONS**------------------
* Safety and effectiveness of Fluzone has not been established in pregnant women. (8.1)
* Antibody responses to Fluzone are lower in persons $\geq$65 years of age than in younger adults. (8.5)

See 17 PATIENT COUNSELING INFORMATION and FDA - approved patient labeling.

Revised: XXXX XXXX

("Fluzone," 2016)

(6)

- The most common (≥10%) local and systemic reactions in children 4 through 8 years of age were pain at the injection site (29%), erythema at the injection site (11%) and fatigue (10%). (6)

- The most common (≥10%) local and systemic reactions in children and adolescents 9 through 17 years of age were pain at the injection site (34%), myalgia (15%), headache (14%) and erythema at the injection site (14%). (6)

To report SUSPECTED ADVERSE REACTIONS, contact Seqirus at 1-855-358-8966 or VAERS at 1-800-822-7967 and www.vaers.hhs.gov.

--------------USE IN SPECIFIC POPULATIONS------------------
- Safety and effectiveness of FLUCELVAX have not been established in pregnant women or nursing mothers. (8.1)
- Geriatric Use: Antibody responses were lower in adults 65 years of age and older than in younger adults. (8.5)

See 17 for PATIENT COUNSELING INFORMATION

Revised: 04/2016

("Flucelvax," 2016)

And finally, any pregnant woman that is given the Fluarix vaccine, should

be enrolled in the pregnancy registry.

The FDA says the pregnancy registry done to monitor for safety and effectiveness of various medications while pregnant. It is worth nothing that the FDA does not monitor or collect data for the registries themselves. Instead, they allow individual companies to monitor themselves. The FDA website says there are 5 vaccine registries for pregnant women, including the flu vaccine, meningitis, and meningococcal vaccines. It is important to note, that the "Mother to Baby" website labels these vaccine registries as "studies." This means that if you are a health care organization requiring mandatory flu shots for your pregnant employees that you must tell them that they are enrolled in a study, and as such, they will be registered with the organization. There is a legal obligation to inform pregnant employees of this fact. Employers must have an "opt out" policy for pregnant employees. And finally, it is the responsibility of the health care organization to let the pregnant woman know that she is being registered with a study and what the pros and cons of such are. The pregnant woman should also have the legal right to opt out of this under the Nuremberg Codes.

During the 2014-2015 flu season, there were 200 pregnant

patients hospitalized for influenza complications ("CDC Influenza

Report," 2015). (It does not appear that a single pregnant patient died of

influenza during this flu season.) It is unethical and medically

unprofessional to mandate that a pregnant woman has an influenza

vaccine. The risks for a pregnant woman and her developing fetus, far

outweigh any potential benefit.

reduce the immune response to FLUVIRIN®.

8   USE IN SPECIFIC POPULATIONS
8.1   Pregnancy
Pregnancy Category B: A reproductive and developmental toxicity study has been
performed in rabbits at a dose level that was approximately 15 times the human dose
based on body weight. The study revealed no evidence of impaired fertility or harm to the
fetus due to FLUVIRIN®. There are, however, no adequate and well-controlled studies in
pregnant women. Because animal reproduction studies are not always predictive of
human response, this vaccine should be used during pregnancy only if clearly needed.

were no vaccine related fetal malformations or other evidence of teratogenicity.

8.3   Nursing Mothers
It is not known whether FLUVIRIN® is excreted in human milk. Because many
drugs are excreted in human milk, caution should be exercised when FLUVIRIN® is
administered to a nursing woman.

8.4   Pediatric Use

("Fluvirin," 2016)

Mask wearing has problems that are immediately apparent. The first is that many of the masks that staff is being forced to wear does not protect them against the influenza virus. The CDC says on their website that they do not recommend that healthy persons wear a mask to prevent transmission of influenza because *"no studies have definitively shown that mask use by either infectious patients or health-care personnel prevents influenza transmission."* The CDC goes on to further state "no recommendation can be made at this time for mask use in the community by asymptomatic persons, including those at high risk for complications, to prevent exposure to influenza" ("Interim Guidance," 2009). This is, in nearly all circumstances, a privacy violation because the use of a mask is being used as a shaming tool and a sign to everyone that the employee is not vaccinated (Papple, 2015).

An area that is never addressed is the ingredients that make up an influenza vaccine. The cell growth of vaccines may be of interest to those who look at vaccine ingredients. Influenza vaccines are "cell based." This means that the vaccine is created by growing the virus in animal cells. The CDC says that these animal cells can be egg or canine kidney cells. The canine kidney cell growth is formally referred to as Madin-Darby Canine Kidney cells, or MDCK ("Cell-Based," 2016). Ingredients of the actual vaccine include, but are not limited to: mercury, formaldehyde, ammonia, canine DNA, phosphates, and various proteins ("Fluzone," 2016; "Flucelvax," 2016).

Employers should take note that the implementation of these policies may be very costly in the long run. Lawsuits have been filed all over the country regarding these policies, and many health care organizations are losing. The EEOC is rapidly jumping in on many of these cases to fight back for the rights of employees.

In Eerie, PA, St. Vincent's hospital was forced to rehire and pay back nearly $300,000 in lost wages to employees they terminated due to a flu shot refusal The EEOC found that the hospital violated the religious rights of the employees, and the employees sued and won. "Saint Vincent implemented the mandatory flu shot policy to receive the maximum reimbursement for treating Medicare patients. At least 95 percent of the hospital's entire workforce had to be vaccinated to meet the requirements, Saint Vincent officials said in 2014 shortly after the policy went into effect. Saint Vincent said in February 2014 that 99.4 percent of its workforce had been vaccinated or received an exemption (Bruce, 2016)." (The link to the actual case can be found here: http://f.datasrvr.com/fr1/216/28078/https-ecf-pawd-uscourts-gov-doc1-15715388813.pdf)

On top of the financial compensation that the hospital will provide in back pay, they will also be responsible for any fines imposed by the EEOC for these violations as well. These fines range from hundreds to thousands of dollars. There are similar lawsuits pending across the United States that the EEOC has filed on behalf of unfairly terminated staff. It will be interesting to see how these cases will transform these policies in the future.

Attorneys are also seeing the increase in employee violations and are quickly jumping on the bandwagon to offer their services to sue employers. This is important to note, because attorney fees, fines, damages, and eventual publicity of the case can cost a hospital system a lot of time and money in legal claims that could be better spent elsewhere.

Clearly, there are financial considerations as well that a hospital must consider. If a hospital is non-profit and they lose money during the reimbursement phase, it could potentially cause them to be displaced, and even shut down. However, the lawsuits that may be filed, the publicity, and the legal fees regarding mandatory vaccine policies should be carefully considered.

The bottom line is that these hospitals and health care systems are not doing this for patient safety. If that was the case, they would also mandate that any patient or visitor coming into their facility have the vaccine. It is being done to pad their pocketbooks, plain and simple. While I understand that a cut in funding can hurt a hospital, they must also look at the fact that they are hurting their own workforce by hiding their policies, and not being fully transparent in the reasons for the mandatory vaccine policies.

It has been suggested that health care workers that choose not to vaccinate for influenza are "stupid," or "uneducated" in their decisions. That they should not be working in health care or should have their license revoked. Nothing could be further from the truth. Health care professionals are some of the most highly educated professionals in the world. They do research every day. They are required to have so many hours of continuing education each year prior to renewing their license. To suggest that these professionals are not able to make good decisions regarding their own health care is insulting at best and frightening at the least. Do you want health care professionals taking care of patients who are not able to safely and soundly make their own medical decisions?

One could also question, if this is now mandatory, what will be next? Forced Bariatric surgery for obese health care workers? Mandatory DNA testing or blood samples to be given? Where will the line be drawn on what an employer can demand of their employees? There is a very slippery rope here that has been oiled, and it should concern everyone that a match may be lit on this one day. Remember, this is not about "patient safety." It's about profit for the hospital and health care system.

Chapter 4

<u>M.D.= Money Doctor?</u>

"Doctors are men who prescribe medicines of which they know little, to cure diseases of which they know less, in human beings of whom they know nothing."

Voltaire

"In the sick room, ten cents' worth of human understanding equals ten dollars' worth of medical science."

Martin H. Fischer

It is no secret that most doctors receive funding (aka "kickbacks") in some way or another from pharmaceutical companies, medical device companies, and even grants from the government. While there have been laws to stop this in recent years, it continues. What *was* secret, up until 2014 was exactly how much your doctor was being "compensated" by these companies. The numerical amounts have been staggering. According to the Centers for Medicare and Medicaid, that number is upwards of $3.5 billion dollars; all for so-called "speaking engagements," "consulting" fees, and even stock ownership in some of the products ("CMS," 2017). The website, if you are interested or curious and want to poke through it, is located at https://www.cms.gov/openpayments/.

The accuracy of this list should be scrutinized. When one searches for doctors who are well known in various communities, and may be even considered famous or infamous, the information can't possibly be correct. I find it very hard to believe that these doctors are not receiving payments of any kind. Some report as little as $35.00. This is highly suspect regarding the accuracy of the data that is being supplied with this list.

It is interesting to note, however, that now that the information is being made public, drug companies are drastically reducing the amount of money they are spending so that they get their product in front of doctors or pay for consulting fees. In 2013, Glaxo Smith Kline reportedly stated that they would no longer be paying any physician to speak on their behalf regarding a product or medication (Thomas, 2013). Novartis, Pfizer, and Eli Lilly have cut their spending on speakers nearly in half since 2011.

Most of these companies have had to settle very large whistleblower lawsuits in the last 10 years over "fraudulent marketing practices." Pfizer was given the one of the largest fines of $2.3 billion dollars in 2009 over fraud for a drug called Bextra (since removed from the market) and for marketing other drugs for off-label uses (Harris, 2009). And in 2013 Johnson and Johnson were given a $3 billion dollar fine over criminal and civil complaint regarding the promotion of Risperdal in unapproved populations (Thomas, 2013). Furthermore, they were also accused of offering kickbacks to prescribing physicians, as well as the pharmacy Omnicare for prescribing this drug to elderly patients, in whom the drug was contraindicated for (Thomas, 2013).

Doctors, while being some of the most highly educated persons on the planet, are also some of the most indebted persons on the planet as well. The average doctor has accrued, on average, $170,000 in student loan debt by the time they graduate (per Google). The average salary for a new physician is right around $210,000 per year (according to a quick Google search). Add on to this the cost of liability insurance at several thousand per year, credentialing costs, CMS penalties, take out taxes, and that doctor is not left with very much money. There is a large burden of financial makeup that the physician must cover to be able to make ends meet, let alone cover the monthly payment for his/her student loans. (In case you're wondering this would come to at least $1000 per month payment, based on a 6% interest rate at 30 years.) Specialists, of course, earn a lot more, but this is looking at what a brand-new physician can expect to make right out of the box.

We have doctors who are up to their eyeballs in debt, pharmaceutical companies that have been involved in numerous fraud cases, and the two want to come together to market and share the love on various products. Does anyone else see a problem with this?

It gets worse.

On top of pharmaceutical companies paying doctors to mislead their patients and the public, we now have insurance companies offering incentive programs to doctors for meeting certain guidelines and protocols. We've all heard about the extremely large number of pediatricians telling parents who choose to not vaccinate, or wish to vaccinate on their own schedule, to take a hike. Ever wondered why? Contrary to the popular claim that it is being done for "the safety of our other patients," there are far more sinister reasons at play.

Some doctors play the "my way or the highway game" like one anonymous physician, (whom I'll call Dr. Narcissist) that posted his story on The Daily Beast on January 2014. He states that "The physician-patient relationship, like so many other human relationships, requires an element of trust. I certainly neither want nor expect a return to the paternalistic "doctor knows best" mindset of bygone years, but I do need to know that patient's parents respect my training and expertise. Refusing an intervention I desperately want all children to receive makes that respect untenably dubious" (Summers, 2014). This "trust" he speaks of is a two-way street.

Why should someone be trusted simply because they have the letters M.D. or D.O. behind their name? Doctors have been known to hurt people, and in some cases, even kill them. The idea that someone should blindly trust another person simply because they have an array of "alphabet soup" behind their name is mind-boggling. And just because he has a diploma on the wall, doesn't mean anything. In October 2015, a man named Rick Van Thiel was charged and arrested with impersonating a doctor, and had a patient caseload of 87. He admitted to having "learned to be a doctor" by watching YouTube videos.

In July 2015, Dr. Christopher Duntsch, a surgeon from Texas, was arrested and charged with "intentionally and knowingly" killing at least four patients.

In 2015, Dr. Farid Fata, a Michigan cancer doctor was sentenced to 45 years in prison after fraudulently and negligently telling patients they had cancer, and then subjected them to expensive treatments and unnecessary pain. (He was paid over $17 million dollars for this by insurance companies and CMS.) And if you don't like these stories, here are a few others where doctors engaged in illegal and unethical behavior to pad their pocketbooks:

"Ricky J. Sayegh, 44, of Scarsdale, New York, pleaded guilty before U.S. District Judge Stanley R. Chesler in Newark federal court to an information charging him with accepting cash bribes in violation of the Federal Travel Act. According to documents filed in this case and statements made in court: Sayegh admitted accepting cash bribes in return for referring blood specimens to BLS. From February 2010 through April 2013, Sayegh received bribes totaling approximately $400,000 from BLS employees and associates. Sayegh's referrals generated more than $1.4 million in lab business for BLS."

"The owner of The Skin Cancer Medical Center in Encino has paid the United States nearly $2.7 million to resolve allegations that he submitted bills to Medicare for Mohs micrographic surgeries for skin cancers that were medically unnecessary. Dr. Norman A. Brooks, M.D., a dermatologist and surgeon, paid the $2,681,400 settlement on April 10."

"Authorities say a Maryland doctor has paid $450,000 to the state to resolve allegations that she submitted false billing records to the Medicaid program. Officials say this week's settlement with Dr. Sabiha Mohiuddin, who owns and operates a primary care practice serving Medicaid patients, stems from a civil complaint filed in the Circuit Court for Frederick County. The complaint alleged that, from January 2007 through February 2014, Mohiuddin billed routine doctor's visits at a higher level of care than was provided to increase reimbursement from the Maryland Medicaid Program."

And these are just a handful of cases in the last couple of years. If you would like to read more about these types of cases and the fraud that is committed in health care each month, then I strongly encourage you to visit the website for the Office of the Inspector General located here: https://oig.hhs.gov/fraud/. The OIG publishes these often and they are updated regularly. Most go ignored in the mainstream media. (All of the above excerpts were taken from the OIG website.)

Not only is it a patient's right to question a doctor, it should be required that all patients are questioning their doctors. They need to check their license status with the state medical board. They need to see that the doctor is not involved in lawsuits. And above all else, they need to see that the doctor has their best interest at heart, and not just his or her pocketbook. Credentialing can find some of this information, but doctors are able to hide their past.

Do you as a patient know how to verify and check out a doctor's license with the medical board? You should. Most, if not all states, have an online registry that you can use to verify this information. It is important to make sure that the doctor that you are seeing is licensed, is not in trouble with the board, and can administer the treatment that you need.

The Patient Bill of Rights also guarantees patients that they have the right to be partners in their health care decisions. This means that patients also get to make decisions; that we don't blindly follow the lead of someone else simply because they tell us to. Any doctor that cannot respect the patient's right to autonomy should not be a physician. The right to informed consent means that we have the right to understand everything- the good and the bad, and then we are to make our determinations and decisions based on that.

Did you know that most "well-child" visits are most often used to vaccinate children? Yes, they measure a child's head circumference and check their weight, but the goal of a well child visit is to vaccinate children. (Whether you choose to do this or not is up to you as a parent, but the fact remains is that vaccination is big money and offers big incentives to physicians, as we will discuss.)

The average cost of a well-child visit is right around $200 (out of pocket or billed to insurance). Add on another $50-75 dollars for immunization charges, and you have on average, a child who is worth about $2500 per year to a physician. If parents didn't need well child visits, and they weren't vaccinating, (or were vaccinated on an alternate schedule) this would drop the child's worth to a physician down to about $500-1000 per year (or less, if the child is relatively healthy). That's a loss of about $1000-1500 per year per child. If a family has four children, that is a loss of up to $6000 per year to that physician. Times this by, say 10 families, and you have now cost that doctor $60,000 per year in fees that he could recoup. No wonder he doesn't want parents questioning his so-called expertise! That could mean a major drop in income for this provider.

Another reason that is rarely discussed by physicians, is that insurance companies have special quotas that they like their physicians to meet. These are called "capitation programs." The insurance companies and physician specialty groups claim that this is done to help reduce health care costs, but the reality is, is that they are incentive programs for physicians. If the doctor can meet these quotas, the insurance companies will offer a "bonus" or "incentive" payment to the physician. Some of these are upwards of $20,000 dollars (Aquire, n.d.). One of the quotas? *Having a required percentage of fully vaccinated pediatric patients.*

This was made extremely apparent in 2016 when a pediatrician group in Livingston, Michigan released the following letter:

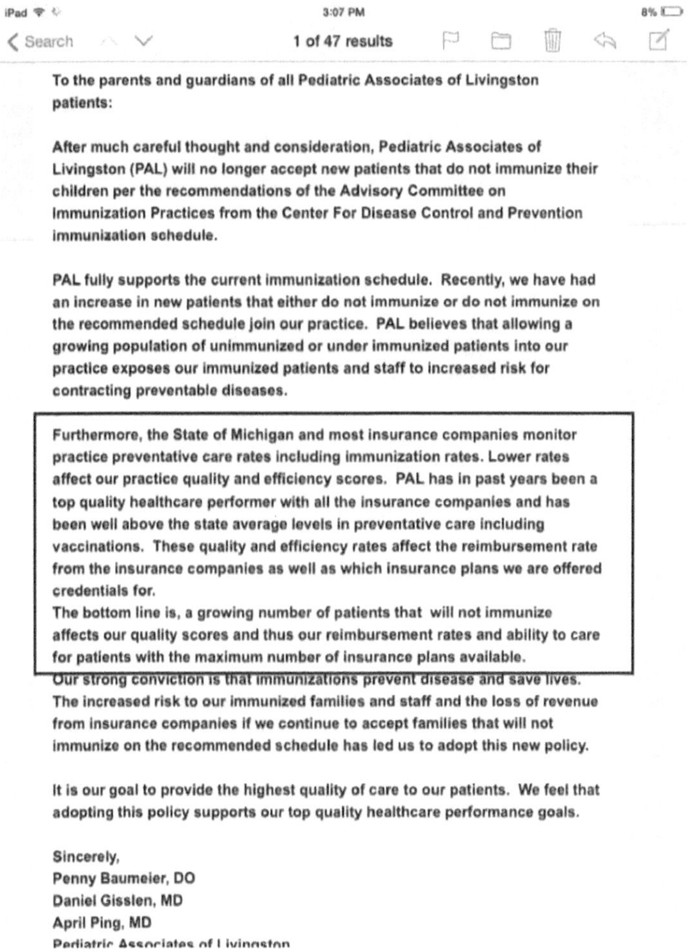

To the parents and guardians of all Pediatric Associates of Livingston patients:

After much careful thought and consideration, Pediatric Associates of Livingston (PAL) will no longer accept new patients that do not immunize their children per the recommendations of the Advisory Committee on Immunization Practices from the Center For Disease Control and Prevention immunization schedule.

PAL fully supports the current immunization schedule. Recently, we have had an increase in new patients that either do not immunize or do not immunize on the recommended schedule join our practice. PAL believes that allowing a growing population of unimmunized or under immunized patients into our practice exposes our immunized patients and staff to increased risk for contracting preventable diseases.

Furthermore, the State of Michigan and most insurance companies monitor practice preventative care rates including immunization rates. Lower rates affect our practice quality and efficiency scores. PAL has in past years been a top quality healthcare performer with all the insurance companies and has been well above the state average levels in preventative care including vaccinations. These quality and efficiency rates affect the reimbursement rate from the insurance companies as well as which insurance plans we are offered credentials for.

The bottom line is, a growing number of patients that will not immunize affects our quality scores and thus our reimbursement rates and ability to care for patients with the maximum number of insurance plans available.

Our strong conviction is that immunizations prevent disease and save lives. The increased risk to our immunized families and staff and the loss of revenue from insurance companies if we continue to accept families that will not immunize on the recommended schedule has led us to adopt this new policy.

It is our goal to provide the highest quality of care to our patients. We feel that adopting this policy supports our top quality healthcare performance goals.

Sincerely,
Penny Baumeier, DO
Daniel Gisslen, MD
April Ping, MD
Pediatric Associates of Livingston

And this is an image from BCBS, the insurance company, demonstrating their capitation program.

HEALTH CARE OUTCOMES: PREVENTIVE HEALTH

CHILDHOOD IMMUNIZATIONS – COMBO 10	
Product lines	**BCN Commercial**
Source	HEDIS
Description	The percentage of children 2 years of age who meet the combination 10 criteria on or before their second birthday: • (4) DTaP* vaccinations • (3) IPV* vaccinations • (1) MMR vaccination • (1) VZV vaccination • (3) HiB* vaccinations • (3) Hepatitis B vaccinations • (4) PCV* vaccinations • (1) HepA vaccination • (2 or 3) RV* vaccinations • (2) Influenza** vaccinations *Vaccinations administered prior to 42 days after birth are not counted as a numerator hit. **Vaccinations administered prior to 180 days after birth are not counted as a numerator hit.
Continuous enrollment	Must be continuously enrolled 12 months prior to child's second birthday
Age criteria	Children who turn 2 years of age during 2016
Exclusionary criteria	Children who are documented with an anaphylactic reaction to the vaccine or its components
Numerator	The number of children who completed vaccinations as defined above
Denominator	The eligible population
Level of measure	Provider level
Target: COMM	63%
Payout: COMM	$400 per Combo 10 completed for each eligible member

Another physician's office has hung this sign up in their offices, and this image was shared in 2017 on social media websites:

> ## NOTIFICATION TO ALL PATIENTS
>
> Bergen West Pediatric Center is notifying you of a service charge of $20.00 for any patient declining vaccine(s) during their scheduled visit with the doctor. If you decline vaccine(s) and wish to spread them out or return at a later date, you will incur this service charge.
>
> The service charge is due to the additional nurses requirements to pull records, verify vaccine(s) and assess the patient.

(One should note that the physician should already have pulled the records, verified patient information and be ready to go prior to seeing the patient. And an internet pull of vaccine records can be useless if a parent or patient has opted out, which they are legally allowed to do. The above is a ploy to inconvenience and penalize those who don't wish to follow the "doctor's orders" and nothing more.)

The American Academy of Pediatrics says that this should not happen:

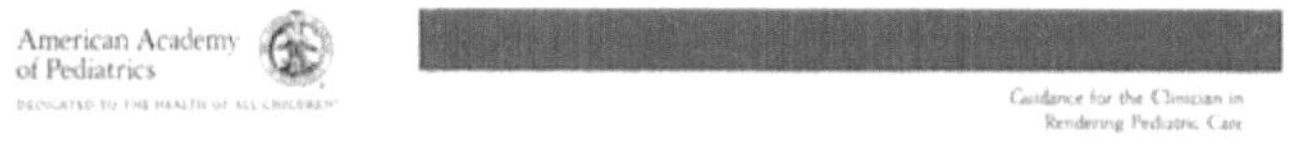

CLINICAL REPORT

Reaffirmation: Responding to Parents Who Refuse Immunization for Their Children

In November 2012, the American Academy of Pediatrics reaffirmed the following publication: Diekema DS, American Academy of Pediatrics, Committee on Bioethics. Responding to parents who refuse immunization for their children. *Pediatrics* 2005;115(5):1428–1431. The reaffirmation includes 1 change in wording, as follows: In the section "Responding to Parents Who Refuse Immunization for Their Children," sixth paragraph, the fifth sentence should read "In general, pediatricians should endeavor not to discharge patients from their practices solely because a parent refuses to immunize a child."

This document is copyrighted and is property of the American Academy of Pediatrics and its Board of Directors. All authors have filed conflict of interest statements with the American Academy of Pediatrics. Any conflicts have been resolved through a process approved by the Board of Directors. The American Academy of Pediatrics has neither solicited nor accepted any commercial involvement in the development of the content of this publication.

The guidance in this report does not indicate an exclusive course of treatment or serve as a standard of medical care. Variations, taking into account individual circumstances, may be appropriate.

("AAP," 2013)

Another area that is just starting to be explored is dentists who are harming small children for profit. One must question why a two-year-old would need multiple root canals on baby teeth. (Particularly when the teeth may be just a few months old themselves.) Unfortunately, some parents are not aware or educated enough to question these procedures, and the dentists completing these procedures are often lying to the parents to get them to agree to the surgery. Some of these children have even died, as they have been given unnecessary dental procedures, and had a cardiac arrest under anesthesia.

One of the best examples of this was in 2007 a story appeared regarding the Small Smiles dentistry chain. Treating children's tooth problems (particularly those with Medicaid) is not profitable for a dentist's office. Undercover investigations found toddlers and small children were tied down and given root canals and other treatment on baby teeth. Sometimes these children didn't speak English, and parents were prohibited from entering the room during treatment (Newhouse, 2010). Ultimately, the company paid a $24 million-dollar settlement and did not admit to any wrong-doing. It appears via a quick Google search, many of these locations are still in practice today.

This practice continues. The problem seems to occur when sedation is used on these pediatric patients. In some cases, it has even caused death.

These are doctors who take an oath to "do no harm." They undertake years and years of schooling to help make and keep you well. Yet these same men and women are willing to sell you and your child out for several thousand dollars a year. This has nothing to do with "keeping patients safe," but everything to do with making sure that they don't lose out on money. Plainly put, it is greed, not patient safety or treatment that is causing many of these policies to be implemented.

Chapter 5

<u>Addiction in America</u>

"No one is immune from addiction; it afflicts people of all ages,

races, classes, and professions."

Patrick J. Kennedy

"It's an addiction... and addiction is something I should know

something about."

Keith Richards

In 2017, the addiction problem in America came to a very ugly

head. People are finally talking about a problem that has been around for

decades, if not a century. One of the biggest problems with the

acknowledgment, however, is the lack of discussion about mental health.

Many addicts self-medicate to treat mental illness. Other problems

include the fact that this has been warned about for years, and the idea

that patients must be satisfied at any cost. There is also an idea that

patients must be "pain free," which has also helped to escalate the

addiction problem.

"When patients visit a doctor's office, outpatient clinic, or hospital, they are often asked to complete a survey rating various aspects of their health care experience. Such surveys may cover many domains, including some outside the ambit of health care, like parking and food service. Where these surveys concern physicians, they usually ask questions about friendliness, responsiveness, and the degree to which the physician inspired confidence and trust. Such patient satisfaction data are playing an increasing role in many important health care decisions. For one thing, physicians can be hired, fired, promoted, and compensated based in part on their patient satisfaction scores. Increasingly, these scores also determine how hospitals are ranked and paid. The Centers for Medicare and Medicaid Services has been publishing this data and has begun distributing funds to hospitals based in part on patient satisfaction" (Gunderman, 2013). Patients are aware of this and have been using this to manipulate and get what they want, and doctors, reluctant to receive a poor score, have been going ahead with prescriptions when they shouldn't have.

In 1986 it was suggested that providing opioids to control pain was "safe and humane" even though the study was done on a minute number of patients (Portenoy & Foley, 1986). Many health care providers took this as a sign and began regularly prescribing copious amounts of opioids for their patients. This, in turn, led to patients demanding the drugs, and doctors simply prescribing them. Unfortunately, many patients were trying to treat emotional pain as if it were physical pain, and they were using pain medications to mask very serious depression, emotional suffering, and other mental health issues.

There is a horrible stigma that comes with having mental health issues today. If you admit to being depressed, anxious, or have other serious mental health issues, you are treated like a pariah. Instead, those with mental health issues tend to self-treat using drugs and alcohol to mask or simply deal with their debilitating symptoms. I believe that this stigma, and the lack of mental health treatment available, is part of what has led to this horrific opioid epidemic. In addiction medicine, these are called co-occurring disorders, and this is the term I will use henceforth. Co-occurring disorders tend to feed off one another. You have emotional pain, some physical pain, and potentially a mental illness, and this can create a monster of a triad for a patient who is struggling (Pohl & Smith, 2012).

"Many patients perceive emotional pain as physical pain and attempt to treat both their physical as well as their emotional pain with opioids. This pattern of coping was first described as "chemical coping" by palliative care specialist Eduardo Bruera, M.D. and colleagues" (Pohl & Smith, 2012). Patients may find that they are able to cope better with everyday life. Before they know it, they are taking the drug in a way that they shouldn't, and they are what is referred to as addicted to the medication. This in turn can cause patients to experience more "physical" pain, and in turn they need a higher dosage of the drug. Unfortunately, these drugs can cause serious adverse effects on the body, which can then cause further issues for the patient short and long term.

This is where things get dicey. Some doctors, instead of sending patients to treatment programs, will continue to prescribe the opioids, and place patients on a "contract" by where the patient signs that they will only take the drug as prescribed, they are subject to pill counts, and they can be dismissed if they violate the rules. This may help protect both doctor and patient, but in the long run, it is not treating the emotional or mental health issues that a patient needs to address to fully assist with the pain that he or she may be experiencing. Doctors that are in the business of pain management, do not want to lose their patients, so they rarely offer mental health treatment as part of the pain management plan. A good pain management doctor will have therapists on board to assist patients in their treatment and diagnosis.

Rehab is an option- but mostly if you have money, or you are willing to live in a homeless shelter type of setting. There is no in-between treatment centers. Most of us have seen the commercials for "Passages of Malibu" or other cushy settings. A few years ago, the television channel VH1 had a show that explored celebrities going through rehab and struggling with addiction. They had nice rooms, recreation, a pool, and excellent food. This is not how most rehabs work for those without money.

The Addiction Center website breaks down the costs of treatment like this:

Detox	Outpatient detox ranges from $1,000 to $1,500 in total. Most inpatient rehabs include detox in the cost of a program. The exact cost of detox depends on whether it's part of an inpatient program and the type of drug addiction being treated. Substances with dangerous detox side effects require more careful monitoring, making the price higher.
Inpatient Rehab	Some inpatient rehabs may cost around $6,000 for a 30-day program. Well-known centers often cost up to $20,000 for a 30-day program. For those requiring 60- or 90-day programs, the total average of costs could range anywhere from $12,000 to $60,000.
Outpatient Rehab	Outpatient programs for mild to moderate addictions are cheaper than inpatient rehab. Many cost $5,000 for a three-month program. Some outpatient programs, such as the program at Hazelden Betty Ford, cost $10,000. The price tag depends on how often the individual visits the center each week and for how long.
Medications	The type of treatment and medications needed affects the price tag on rehab. Some people don't need medication for their addiction. Medications most often treat alcohol and opiate addiction. It can cost several thousand dollars a year. Year-long methadone treatment for heroin users costs around $4,700.

(Addiction Center, n.d.)

Some insurances will pay for some alcohol and drug treatment, but again, there are problems with this. Insurances often require prior authorization. Most addicted patients hide this from a doctor and getting a prior authorization can be time consuming and lengthy. Many addiction treatment centers do not have enough beds, and there can be wait lists for those seeking treatment.

There is also the use of methadone in the treatment of addiction. Some believe that this is simply replacing one drug for another. Others argue that due to the regulation and required counseling, mandatory random drug screens, and low cost, that this is a great option for those who truly wish to seek help (AddictionInfo, 2010). Suboxone is another low-cost treatment option for those struggling with addiction, but few doctors can prescribe it, due to federal regulations that accompany the use of the medication.

Many who struggle with addiction and mental illness are poor, underserved, of a minority population, and simply do not have the resources with which to obtain treatment. Many mental health facilities throughout the United States have been shuttered due to budget cuts and other funding issues. There is also a lack of mental health providers in the country. Patients often end up visiting emergency rooms, urgent care centers, or they are wait-listed for months at a time before they can receive treatment (Ochoa, 2017). The funding is not available, and even if it were, the treatment options available are few and far between.

What can be done about this? Some states via their attorney generals have taken it upon themselves to sue the pharmaceutical companies. "The complaints typically allege the wholesale distributors violated the federal Controlled Substances Act by failing to alert the U S Drug Enforcement Administration of suspicious opioids purchases, such as orders of unusual size, frequency or pattern. The claims against the manufacturers are based on allegations the companies exaggerated the benefits of the medication and knew the drugs were being overly prescribed, yet failed to warn doctors of the extremely addictive nature of the narcotics and the need to strictly limit the dose" ("Levin Law," n.d.)

Other states, such as Nevada, have made strict prescribing laws. Starting in January of 2018, they required mandatory education on opioid prescribing, maximum dosing guidelines, and checking the state registry for cross-prescriptions. It is very thorough and very detailed.

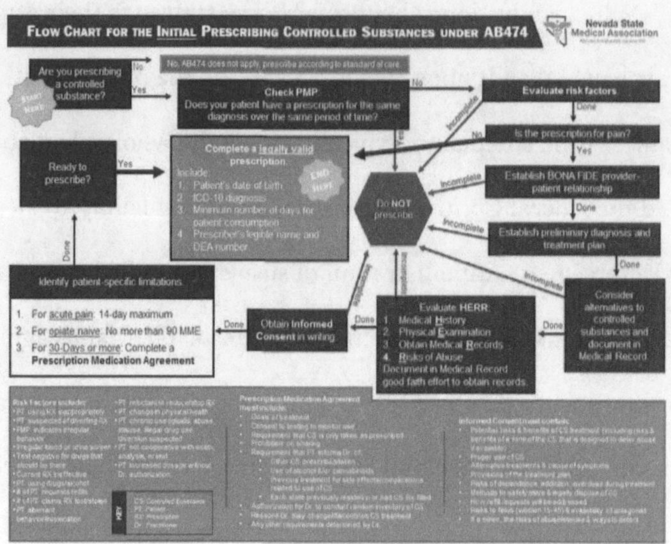

(https://nvdoctors.org/practice-resources/prescribing-opioids/)

This is fine; financially punish those who have helped in the creation of this problem. However, it does not address the real problems; a scarlet letter for mental illness, lack of funding, and lack of access to drug and alcohol treatment and treatment for mental illness. This witch hunting is only going to service as a façade for dealing with the real problem. There is no real solution as to what will happen if the states win their cases. Why not set up a type of fund that will help those with addiction or mental illness should they win their case?

It remains to be seen what will come of this serious problem. One thing is clear, and that is America needs better access to mental health, and addiction treatment. We must stop belittling those who wish to receive treatment for mental illness. Doctors need to stop prescribing pain medication to treat emotional pain, because it is not working. And we need to put funding toward getting better mental health care in this country before it's too late.

Chapter 6

<u>Pharma and the Professor/Fraud in Research</u>

"Conflicts of interest and financial relationships between drug companies are ubiquitous in almost every single aspect of medical practice and medical research and medical education in the U.S."

Eric Campbell

"Scientific fraud, plagiarism, and ghost writing are increasingly being reported in the news media, creating the impression that misconduct has become a widespread and omnipresent evil in scientific research."

Heinrich Rohrer

Higher education is no exception to being purchased and bought out by pharmaceutical companies. In 2009, the New York Times blew the lid off a hidden secret that was always sort of talked about but never really discussed. In the article, the Times raised serious issues of conflict of interest in higher education. "In a first-year pharmacology class at Harvard Medical School, Matt Zerden grew wary as the professor promoted the benefits of cholesterol drugs and seemed to belittle a student who asked about side effects. Mr. Zerden later discovered something by searching online that he began sharing with his classmates. The professor was not only a full-time member of the Harvard Medical faculty, but a paid consultant to 10 drug companies, including five makers of cholesterol treatments" (Wilson, 2009).

Just a few months later, Harvard issued their university- wide policy on "Financial Conflicts of Interest" ("Conflict," n.d.). Unfortunately, a mere six years later, that has been relaxed, and Harvard now allows conflicts of interest to occur, all in the name of "potentially saving lives" (my quote not necessarily theirs) (Bailey, 2016). If this type of issue is occurring at prestigious institutions, it must be occurring at other, smaller, institutions, right? The resounding answer is yes!

One of the best sources for finding out more information on a school's conflict of interest, when it comes to financial compensation from pharmaceutical companies, is the American Medical Student Association (AMSA). The AMSA offers a fully transparent grading and rating system on their website to demonstrate schools that are in violation of the policies, and those that hold themselves to a higher accountability. Some of the worst offenders? Rutgers, Duke, Touro University, and Michigan State among others. This information, however, is not complete. Not all schools have conflict of interest policies, and not all schools require disclosure. This website can offer a small insight into what faculty are receiving "gifts" but it doesn't show the whole picture. You can learn more about this website here: http://amsascorecard.org/.

Some may ask, "why is this a problem?" because the answer may not be clear. Keep in mind that many of these professors are tenured. They receive lucrative salaries and benefits. On top of that, many are in prestigious circles of influence and wealth. When a professor also has helped to develop a drug, and then pushes this drug on his/her students for them to hand out to patients later, this is clearly a conflict of interest. The professor may not only be getting a payment from the pharmaceutical company (stock, cash, bonus, etc.) but they may be getting speaking fees, book writing fees, grants, and other compensation when they are able to "sell" their drug. We rely on doctors/physicians to be honest, but can they truly be transparent when they have a financial interest in the subject matter that they are teaching to impressionable minds? I believe that answer is no.

Students have also reported being censored in many cases with their projects and research that may conflict with the "official" (aka "paid) stance of the university.

Misconduct. Deceit. Dishonesty. Hustle. Racket. Plagiarism. Con. Call it what you want, but fraud is fraud, and it is rampant in research. In 2016 authors Kearns, Schmidt, and Glantz reported that this is not only a long-term problem, but it is still occurring. Their study explored the impact that the sugar industry has had on research and findings. They determined that the sugar industry, starting in the 60's funded research to show that sugar had no effect on Coronary Heart Disease, and they conclude their study by stating: "Because CHD is the leading cause of death globally, the health community should ensure that CHD risk is evaluated in future risk assessments of added sugars. Policymaking committees should consider giving less weight to food industry–funded studies and include mechanistic and animal studies as well as studies appraising the effect of added sugars on multiple CHD biomarkers and disease development." What does this mean? It means that money speaks, and payment is being exchanged in return for fraudulent studies being published.

The real question, is why is this happening? Well, first and foremost, money is the biggest factor. Billions of dollars across many industries are always at stake. Anytime there is a statement that something causes cancer, or disease, or heart attack, it is all over the media. This results in negative publicity for a company or organization. Using the sugar industry for example, the purchase of soft drinks has been down every year for the last decade (Kell, 2016).

In academia, there is a push for all faculty to be published (Herndon, 2016). Herndon suggests: "With publication in top-tier journals now requisite for advancement within academia as universities and even some countries attempt to use publications in top-tier journals to upgrade their image, the pressure to publish has never been greater. Even in universities without a research culture (often called "teaching" schools to contrast with more research-focused "research" schools) where heavy teaching loads are the norm, requirements for publication are being added even though there is no institutional support for research (e.g., research funding; research-trained doctoral students; release time from teaching loads to conduct research; and appropriate library print, digital, and online resources). The professors, trained as teachers with only a light research basting, have very limited research skills and research experience. Perhaps unethical research shortcuts are inevitable in these unsupportive environments as the risk of detection may be small compared with the certainty of dismissal and a difficult job hunt if papers are not published." Professors who complete research are also able to assist in getting the University monetary grants; this can strengthen a candidate's standing regarding achieving tenure. This again, boils down to money.

Tenure is a very big deal at a university. In many cases it appears it is a permanent employment placement. This is not what tenure was supposed to be. "One major concern with the tenure system is that granting tenure can lead to unproductive faculty members. Once a faculty member has achieved tenure and has been promoted, the incentive to perform at a high level may be significantly reduced. In fact, the tenure system may promote complacency and allow faculty members to underachieve while leaving the institution no recourse. In addition, tenured faculty members are the highest paid faculty members, leaving universities with less money to hire new faculty members and adjust to the changing academic climate. Tenure is a long-term commitment of the institution to a faculty member. 18 With the age limit for retirement being eliminated by the Age Discrimination in Employment Act, tenured faculty members technically never have to retire. It is a guaranteed job for life with no guarantee of productivity" (Asbill et al., 2016, p. 4).

When staff are encouraged to get published, unfortunately, fraud can also occur. Fraud doesn't just occur in academia, but at many levels of the scientific community via peer review systems. The system of peer review is fraught with problems. Südhof (2016) suggests that there are three problems with peer review: hidden conflict of interest, little to no accountability, and no competition in journals for communicating new sciences.

Another problem with peer review, is competition. Competition can be for jobs, placements, grants, funding, and even speaking engagements. If a peer reviewer was/is competing for one of the same incentives that an author is working for, is this ethical? Balietti, Goldstone, and Helbing (2016) observed "competition proved to be a double-edged sword: on the one hand, it fosters innovation and product diversity, but on the other hand, it also leads to more unfair reviews and to a lower level of agreement between reviewers." Does this allow for companies, and even the public to receive fair and unbiased information? Balietti, Goldstone, and Helbing's findings would suggest that the answer to this would be no.

There are many examples of peer review fraud. In 2014 engineer Peter Chen had 60 articles retracted because he faked over 130 email addresses to provide fraudulent peer reviews of his writings (Haug, 2015).

It has been shown that there is also purposeful fraud being committed in research. Hundreds of papers have been redacted over the years due to purposeful fraud. Steen's report in 2011 concluded that "the results suggest that papers retracted because of data fabrication or falsification represent a calculated effort to deceive. It is inferred that such behaviour is neither naïve, feckless nor inadvertent."

What happens when a paper gets retracted? This means it gets pulled from publication. However, some studies suggest that it can take anywhere from 3-5 years before this happens. And sometimes, it never happens at all; some publications allow people to make corrections and then resubmit the manuscript as if nothing ever happened.

Then we have the redactions themselves. Sometimes they are nothing more than a witch hunt. Probably, and arguably, the most famous retraction was Dr. Andrew Wakefield's paper in 1998, that "linked the MMR with autism." The fact is, is that the paper that Dr. Wakefield et al. released, never said that. It never said anything close to that. This study that for years was reported as such a fraud stated, and I quote, "We did not prove an association between measles, mumps, and rubella vaccine and the syndrome described. Virological studies are underway that may help to resolve this issue." The study concluded by stating: "We have identified a chronic enterocolitis in children that may be related to neuropsychiatric dysfunction. In most cases, onset of symptoms was after measles, mumps, and rubella immunisation. *Further investigations are needed to examine this syndrome and its possible relation to this vaccine*" (Wakefield et al., 1998). You can read the full text of the retracted study here: http://www.thelancet.com/journals/lancet/article/PIIS0140-6736(97)11096-0/fulltext. (The emphasis here is that of this author.)

I use the example of Wakefield to demonstrate that even if research may be qualified, it may get pulled if it "rocks the boat" or the status quo. (Which, with the MMR vaccine, all hell broke loose when profits started to diminish, and people started to question the vaccine's safety.) It is interesting to note, that a study released in 2017 suggests that gut health is tied to brain diseases, which is ultimately what Wakefield et al. explored as well. The study released by the University of Pennsylvania School of Medicine (2017) concluded that "bacteria in the gut microbiome drive the formation of cerebral cavernous malformations (CCMs), clusters of dilated, thin-walled blood vessels in the brain that can cause stroke and seizures." Recent studies also suggest that Alzheimer's, is also connected to gut health and it demonstrates that there is a link between poor gut health and effects on the brain (Rong & QuanQiu, 2016).

The witch hunts that have occurred to those who dare expose various nefarious practices are nothing new. Many scientists have had their careers ruined by exposing the truth and by questioning the status quo. Walter Nelson-Rees was one such researcher who had this experience.

"Exposing contaminated cell lines cost Walter Nelson-Rees his career. He was an expert in culturing human and animal cells at the University of California, Berkeley, and ran a cell line bank in Oakland. From 1975 to 1981, he published a series of articles in Science outing contaminated lines and naming the laboratories where they had originated. His angry colleagues called his publications a "hit list." In an editorial, Nature's editor-in-chief, John Maddox, railed against "self-appointed vigilantes." Nelson-Rees' work made it clear that HeLa contamination was far from the only problem. Eventually, the NIH terminated his contract, and he became so isolated from his peers that he left science and became an art dealer" (Neimark, 2014).

A large area that appears to be problematic is the fact that a lot of peer reviewed studies can't be replicated when another scientist or research team tries to duplicate the results. This may suggest a worrying trend that fraudulent studies are being pushed through (Feilden, 2017). Replicating studies can be time-consuming and costly, and many studies are not duplicated for these reasons. If a reviewer does not choose to replicate, should they be held liable if the study shows itself to be fraudulent? This is one of the many ideas that have been introduced in recent years due to the increase in fraud in research studies.

What qualifies a peer reviewer to be a peer reviewer? Well, that depends on the publication. Every single publication has its own requirements for a person to qualify as a peer reviewer. In most cases, peer reviewers are volunteers. They are told to be truthful, critical, ethical, and confidential. They are also peers of those who are submitting articles, writings, and research (Jacobson et al., 2017). Clearly, these guidelines are not always followed, as I have shown in the above examples.

I was recently speaking with another colleague of mine, and we discussed these various scenarios. We talked about the fraud that is continuing today, and how big of an influence money is. One of the biggest problems is that we cannot have true science unless we forego influence and allow scientists to conduct research and find new evidence-based practices in medicine. However, we cannot complete research and work to find new and real scientific breakthroughs without financial funding. It is a horrible Catch-22.. How do we go about funding without political, corporate, or other groups swaying scientific findings? It is nearly impossible in the current climate.

Something must change. We have those continuing to say "the science is settled" but how can science ever be settled? New findings pop up continuously. How can science be settled if there is a financial or a corporate conflict of interest? It can't. We must find new ways to approach science without influence if we wish to go back to true scientific discovery. Even if the science contradicts what financial backers wish for the science to say. You cannot have true progress unless you allow science to truly be investigated and researched.

Chapter 7

<u>Mass Media, Big Pharma, and Drug Prices</u>

"Every night I watch the nightly news. It's funded by the pharmaceutical companies. Virtually every ad is a drug ad. They get their say every night on the nightly news through advertising."

Michael Moore

"Since 1994, lawmakers on both sides of the aisle have considered it politically risky to offer a plan to fix America's broken health care system. The American public, though, has paid the price for this silence as health care costs skyrocketed, millions went uninsured, and millions more grappled with financial insecurity and hardship."

Ron Wyden

Turn on the television to the nightly news, and you are likely to be inundated with medical advertisements, prescription drugs, and vaccination commercials. The reason for this is simple: pharmaceutical companies invest heavily in the media to spread awareness about a drug and to advertise their drugs and medical procedures. They do this in hopes that patient Bob will make an appointment with his doctor and request the medication listed. These same pharmaceutical companies have also created a large part of the problem with the narcotic and addiction issues that we have in this country.

Open any magazine on the shelves today and you will find copious amounts of pharmaceutical advertisements. In fact, I pulled apart one recent magazine and found a half-dozen pharmaceutical advertisements inside. Journals sent to medical professionals are full of pharmaceutical advertisements each month as well.

The cost of medications in the last thirty years has absolutely skyrocketed. One of the earliest examples of this happening in recent years was when AZT was released for AIDS patients in the late 1987 and it cost between $8000-$12000 per year, per patient. At the time, it was the most expensive medication ever placed on the market. (It was estimated that the company producing AZT would stand to make upwards of $250 million per year.) In 2017, $8000 per year medications are considered cheap in comparison ("AZT," 1989).

In the last two years, outrage has been raised over Martin Shkreli raising the price of a medication to $750 per pill. The makers of Epi-pen, Mylan, reported record profits after they raised the prices of the pens to over $600, and cutting their generic partner out of production. Both drugs in question are life-saving drugs (Bomey, 2016). Some schools across the country are also now required to have Epi-pens available and must train staff on how to use them. Coincidence? Nah.

One must also examine the high cost of drugs such as insulin. Insulin has been on the market for nearly 1oo years. Why, then, does a bottle for a month supply cost anywhere from $200-$600? Shouldn't they have perfected a medication like this by now? After all, aspirin and acetaminophen are sold for pennies. Why not insulin? Why are patients who are struggling to pay their bills having to decide between their life-saving medications and paying the heating bill? The simple answer: money (Kelto, 2015).

Drug companies can change a single molecule of a formula and re-patent any medication like insulin. These are referred to as "biosimilars." For example: "Lilly and Boehringer Ingelheim's biosimilar version of glargine was recently approved in the European Union. In the United States, the same product received tentative approval from the Food and Drug Administration, but final approval is being held up for 30 months, until mid-2016, because Sanofi has filed a lawsuit claiming patent infringement" (Tucker, 2015)

Some doctors have resorted to telling their patients to request a vial for "their dog" at the vet, which can cost around $20-25, and to use that insulin, because it is identically the same as the insulin that they use. Something is very wrong with this picture.

Another medication that has gone up significantly in recent years is albuterol- an inhaler for those with asthma and breathing problems. A group of Congressmen and women looked at the increase in various drug prices in 2014, and what they found was alarming as to the rate of increase. You can view the complete compilation here:

https://www.sanders.senate.gov/download/face-sheet-on-generic-drug-price-increases?inline=file

Drug	Use	Average Market Price Oct. 2013	Average Market Price April 2014	Average Percentage Increase
Doxycycline Hyclate (bottle of 500, 100 mg tablets)	antibiotic used to treat a variety of infections	$20	$1,849	8,281%
Albuterol Sulfate (bottle of 100, 2 mg tablets)	used to treat asthma and other lung conditions	$11	$434	4,014%
Glycopyrrolate (box of 10 0.2 mg/mL, 20 mL vials)	used to prevent irregular heartbeats during surgery	$65	$1,277	2,728%
Divalproex Sodium ER (bottle of 80, 500 mg tablets ER 24H)	used to prevent migraines and treat certain types of seizures	$31	$234	736%

The drug market cannot continue to sustain itself as is. People are having to choose between heating their homes, paying rent, and affording to stay alive by taking medications. Others are not taking the medications properly or are taking them as they see fit in hopes that a little at a time will help them, rather than taking the medication as prescribed. It is a recipe for disaster as the Baby Boomer Generation begins to enter its senior citizen years.

Some may ask, "Well, what about buying meds online?" or "I hear people order meds from Canada all of the time." Anyone who has traveled overseas knows that medications are drastically cheaper than in the United States. In some cases, some drugs are even available over the counter. This may seem like a solution for some, but it may land you in prison ("Centers," n.d.).

The FDA further warns that there are risks to buying online-namely they state the "high level of quality assurance" found in the USA, but they don't mention that it also bites into the profits of the doctors and the pharmaceutical companies who supply these costs here in the United States versus Canada or Mexico. There is no reason why a medication can be sold over the border in Canada for $15.00 but for $1500 here in the United States; it is simply absurd.

Senior citizens must worry yearly about the annual so-called "donut hole." If you aren't aware of what this is, it is a drug coverage gap for patients on Medicare. It places a limit on what a company will pay for a drug for a certain period. Patients then must pay out of pocket for a drug until the insurance payments will kick back in. It is financially devastating people each year and drains the financial resources of many seniors ("CMS," n.d.). Some seniors end up paying thousands of dollars out of pocket for their medications simply to stay alive. There are so-called "Extra Help" programs available from CMS, but the guidelines for these are strict, and very few people qualify for them.

One must also question if most of the medications prescribed are truly necessary for many of these patients. Does a patient really need to be on 5 blood pressure medications? Does a 100-year-old patient in a nursing home need to be on 15 different medications? (I have personally seen this!)

"The statistics on medication usage among elderly patients in the US are eye-opening: more than one-third of prescription drugs used in the US are taken by elderly patients; the ambulatory elderly fill between 9-13 prescriptions a year (including new prescriptions and refills); the average elderly patient is taking more than five prescription medications; the average nursing home patient is taking seven medications" ("How Many," 2010).

One study on geriatrics and medications showed the following data: "At the age of 100, 73% of individuals (79% of women, 54% of men) had received one or more prescription drugs, with a median of 7 (interquartile range 0–12) prescription items. The most frequently prescribed drug classes were cardiovascular (53%), central nervous system (CNS) (53%), and gastrointestinal (47%). Overall, 32% of participants (28% of men, 32% of women) who received drug prescriptions may have received one or more potentially inappropriate prescriptions, with temazepam and amitriptyline being the most frequent. CNS prescriptions were potentially inappropriate in 23% of individuals, and anticholinergic prescriptions were potentially inappropriate in 18% of individuals" (Hazra et al., 2016).

It should also be taken into consideration that taxpayers are paying for most of these medications. While I do not begrudge our elderly and our seniors for needing health care and medications, I do have to wonder if we aren't harming them more than helping them with the amount of medications that are clearly being over prescribed to this at-risk population. Particularly when this generation of the elderly has been taught not to question doctors and to do as they are told. It creates a somewhat indelicate situation. One must wonder who is protecting the potentially unprotected?

Chapter 8

<u>The "Satisfied" Patient</u>

"When Department of Health and Human Services administrators decided to base 30 percent of hospitals' Medicare reimbursement on patient satisfaction survey scores, they likely figured that transparency and accountability would improve health care."

Alexandra Robbins

Without beating around the bush, let me come right out and say that patient satisfaction surveys are killing health care and are potentially killing the patients they were intended to protect. They have become a huge part of the problem and a huge detriment to quality care. Since the implementation of these surveys, it has been made clear that patients have the control in the health care setting. While this does help promote self-advocacy, it also creates a conflict when it comes to medical professionals determining what the best course of action for a patient is. Patients now have the "control", if you will, but this so-called power has not come without a steep cost to quality of care, and the potential of death to the patient.

Providers, both Doctors and Advanced Practitioners, have many years of medical training. They are also knowledgeable and have been tested with high and rigorous standards. They attended school for many years and have had residencies and clinical hours to prove their capabilities to treat and handle patients. Yet we ask those who may not even have a high school education, and who may or may not be able to read and write, to rate the care that is given to them based on many varying factors. (i.e. Was your pain "controlled?")

The primary survey used for patients is called the Hospital Consumer Assessment of Health care Providers and Systems (aka HCAHPS). Per the Centers for Medicare and Medicaid: "The HCAHPS Survey is composed of 27 items: 18 substantive items that encompass critical aspects of the hospital experience (communication with doctors, communication with nurses, responsiveness of hospital staff, cleanliness of the hospital environment, quietness of the hospital environment, pain management, communication about medicines, discharge information, overall rating of hospital, and recommendation of hospital); four items to skip patients to appropriate questions; three items to adjust for the mix of patients across hospitals; and two items to support congressionally-mandated reports" ("CMS FAQ," n.d.).

The HCAHPS survey is used nationwide to determine care, and reports are completed quarterly on the CMS website in reporting the findings and the results of the surveys in comparison. Any person who has access to the internet can view these reports.

"Beginning in October 2012, the Affordable Care Act implemented a policy withholding 1 percent of total Medicare reimbursements—approximately $850 million—from hospitals (that percentage will double in 2017). Each year, only hospitals with high patient-satisfaction scores and a measure of certain basic care standards will earn that money back, and the top performers will receive bonus money from the pool (Robbins, 2015)."

There are many problems with patients judging their satisfaction and the level of care that they receive. One of the biggest problems, are safety issues. Patients who report a "higher patient satisfaction was associated with less emergency department use but with greater inpatient use, higher overall health care and prescription drug expenditures, and increased mortality (Fenton et al., 2012)." In other words, the happier a patient is with the care, the more likely he or she is to remain unhealthy, and even die because of the high level of satisfaction.

Perhaps you are a patient reading this. Did you know that if you complain, let's say, about not getting sugar with your coffee on your satisfaction survey, a nurse is likely to be punitively punished for this, and have this placed in his/her personnel file? Or, let's say that you complain that your pain wasn't controlled to your liking. The doctor that prescribed pain meds is likely to get reprimanded or perhaps even fired. Why? Because your complaints and "lack of satisfaction" are tied directly to the hospital's reimbursement (Gunderman, 2013) if you are using Medicare or Medicaid.

CMS of course, claims that this does not happen (which you can see based on the slide presentation they put out here: **https://www.qualityreportingcenter.com/wp-content/uploads/2016/01/IQR-VBP_HCAHPS-and-Pain-Management_20160128_vFINAL508.pdf**). They also claim that they do not encourage opioid use. However, most patients believe that "pain control" means "no pain" and by asking patients if their pain was controlled, they are setting up hospitals and health care providers for failure by asking questions such as these.

The following is a letter published by the American Hospital Association regarding pain management questions. (The letter can be found here: http://www.aha.org/advocacy-issues/letter/2016/160428-let-hcahps.pdf.) I believe this letter speaks for itself:

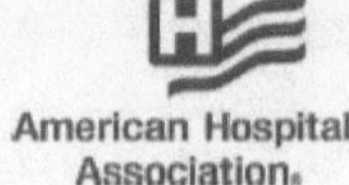

American Hospital Association®

800 10th Street, NW
Two CityCenter, Suite 400
Washington, DC 20001-4956
(202) 638-1100 Phone
www.aha.org

April 28, 2016

Sean Cavanaugh
Deputy Administrator and Director
Center for Medicare
Centers for Medicare & Medicaid Services
7500 Security Boulevard, Room 305H.2.
Baltimore, MD 21244

RE: HCAHPS pain questions

Dear Mr. Cavanaugh:

On behalf of our nearly 5,000 member hospitals, health systems and other health care organizations, and our 43,000 individual members, I am writing to you about concerns that the Hospital Consumer Assessment of Healthcare Providers and Services (HCAHPS) survey questions related to pain management may inadvertently be contributing to the opioid epidemic. We were pleased to hear you say during the February 24 Senate Special Committee on Aging hearing that the Centers for Medicare & Medicaid Services (CMS) has research underway to determine whether there is a better way to ask these questions.

The AHA appreciates your willingness to reassess the pain questions to address these concerns and urges you to complete this review quickly. As your work progresses, we look forward to providing hospital leaders' perspective about the need to reframe the questions. In the meantime, we ask CMS to suspend the three pain-related questions in the Value-Based Purchasing (VBP) Program.

Our members see the harm caused by opioid addiction, and they appreciate the many steps the Administration is taking to support providers and first responders as they work to save lives. We believe that a review and redesign of these pain questions is aligned with other important actions the Administration is taking to stop the epidemic, such as developing opioid prescribing guidelines for chronic pain; proposing regulatory changes, as well as allocating funding, to expand access to medication-assisted treatment; and approving the life-saving drug Narcan as a nasal spray.

There are currently three questions about pain management in the HCAHPS survey. The first question, "During this hospital stay, did you need medicine for pain?", may imply to patients that medication is the best or only way to address pain. The second question asks, "During this hospital stay, how often was your pain well controlled?" The third question is particularly concerning, because it asks, "During this hospital stay, how often did the hospital staff do *everything they could* to help you with your pain?" (emphasis added).

Linking the pain control questions to payment through the VBP program is seen by clinicians as encouragement from CMS to provide pain medication, even if the questions ultimately represent a small portion of a hospital's performance score. Suspending the questions will send a clear signal that CMS does not want to create an expectation that pain management should always include use of powerful prescription drugs such as opioids. The AHA agrees that the HCAHPS survey should inquire about pain management, that performance scores should be publicly reported, and that redesigned pain questions should eventually be reincorporated into the VBP program. **However, we also want to ensure that the questions do not create pressure to prescribe opioids or other prescription painkillers or punish providers who, in their best judgment, choose not to prescribe them.**

The opioid epidemic has taken a staggering toll. At the same time, we recognize that the under-treatment of pain can have a significant impact on individuals' health and quality of life. As the health care field works to ensure that patients are neither undertreated for pain nor overprescribed opioids, the AHA welcomes the opportunity to work with CMS in designing and pilot testing alternative questions. We have reached out to agency staff to express our willingness to support this effort, and we look forward to a continued dialogue.

If you have further questions, please contact Nancy Foster, vice president of quality and patient safety policy, at nfoster@aha.org, or Evelyn Knolle, senior associate director of policy, at eknolle@aha.org.

Sincerely,

/s/

Ashley Thompson
Senior Vice President
Public Policy Analysis and Development

Staff are and will continue to be punished for poor scores if

questions such as these remain in the patient satisfaction surveys.

It is very safe to say that many patients are not legally or professionally qualified to be rating the care that they receive. Many patients are quite ill when they are presented in a health care facility. They may also be heavily drugged and more than a little "out of it." With that in mind, appearances may not be as they seem. They may have false memories and may not have full facts when they are filling out surveys. They may also have family members influencing what is said.

The patient satisfaction survey administrators, of course, don't want to lose this gravy train. In fact, one executive, regularly tells doctors and providers to "suck it up" (Falkenberg, 2013). Survey companies have nothing to lose of course, except a lot of money should health care systems and facilities decide to shut down these problem-child survey systems. Studies show that the more satisfied a patient is, the more likely they are to die. Survey companies such as Press Ganey say that patients are more satisfied because a provider is attempting to prevent malpractice by over-prescribing and over-testing (Falkenberg, 2013). (While there may be some truth to this, the truth of the matter is, these surveys can kill a provider's career. They want the patient satisfied at all costs.)

"The math is now simple for doctors: More tests and stronger drugs equal more satisfied patients, and more satisfied patients equal more pay. The biggest loser: the patient, who may not receive appropriate care. … These ethical dilemmas are playing out across the country, with the need to please customers often trumping their health. In a recent online survey of 700-plus emergency room doctors by Emergency Physicians Monthly, 59% admitted they increased the number of tests they performed because of patient satisfaction surveys. The South Carolina Medical Association asked its members whether they'd ever ordered a test they felt was inappropriate because of such pressures, and 55% of 131 respondents said yes. Nearly half said they'd improperly prescribed antibiotics and narcotic pain medication in direct response to patient satisfaction surveys" (Falkenberg, 2013).

Another problem lies in the fact that the surveys are not necessarily accurate. Press Ganey admitted that they need at least 30 to draw quality data from these, yet they routinely deliver results that often may only be 8-10 responses per month. This also means that providers are not receiving real tracking data, and neither is the government, or tax paying citizens for that matter. CMS is the primary group that sets standards for care, and CMS is the organization that has reimbursement rates tied to care standards (Falkenberg, 2013). How they can determine this based on skewed or incomplete data, reeks of fraud. (Ultimately HCAHPS has replaced Press Ganey, but the questions are still the same, as are the scenarios used in the questions.)

Patients need to be able to provide feedback in a constructive manner. However, patient satisfaction surveys that are tied to reimbursement are not the way to accomplish this. Open dialogue, better patient education, and better communication between staff and patients is the best way to approach a more open and honest patient experience in the health care setting.

Chapter 9

Data Mining and Selling of Your Medical Records

Even though people pretend that medical records are privileged information, anyone can already get their hands on them.
Craig Venter

One new area that has popped up in the last five years is the data mining and reselling of individual private medical information. For this chapter, I am not even sure where to begin, except to start by saying that there are companies popping up every single day and night that are purchasing your private medical information and selling it to employers, life insurance companies, health insurance companies, and anyone who may have a vested interest in your private medical information- and 90% of people are not even aware that this is going on. I learned about this information at the very last minute and decided to include a last chapter to discuss this horrifying movement.

Has your employer started a "biometric screening" process to lower your health insurance rates? These biometric screenings get your height, weight, blood sugar, blood pressure, cholesterol, and offer you "counseling" if your numbers are not where they should be. If you pass, you may get a good savings on your health insurance each year. Some employers require intensive counseling and weight loss programs, and other medical visits if you don't pass. And if you don't lose weight, drop cholesterol, etc. you may still be penalized in your insurance premiums. Supposedly, this is all done to save both the employer and the employee money, but at what cost? Approximately 50% of large health care firms have made these biometric screenings required or mandatory of their employers, and this number continues to grow. Some employees are even finding themselves without a job if they refuse the wellness biometric screenings.

There are minimal savings to employers using these. The ACA puts limits on the incentive percentage that an employer can receive for these. Yes, it may lower costs, but what these programs are really set up for, is to make sure you are compliant, or you can be discriminated against with higher health insurance costs. Conveniently, the ACA does not address collection practices on this information.

The EEOC suggests that this is a potentially huge area where ADA violations can occur. Per the EEOC: "Title I of the ADA is a federal civil rights law that prohibits employers from discriminating against individuals on the basis of disability. It also generally restricts employers from obtaining medical information from applicants and employees, but allows them to make inquiries about employees' health or do medical examinations that are part of a voluntary employee health program. Employee health programs include many workplace wellness programs.

Additionally, Title I of the ADA prohibits employers from denying employees access to wellness programs based on disability and requires employers to provide reasonable accommodations (adjustments or modifications) that allow employees with disabilities to participate in wellness programs and to keep any medical information gathered as part of the wellness program confidential" ("EEOC," n.d.).

Chances are, you have okayed this without even realizing it. When you are signing your rights away, or singing a privacy information sheet, often these types of data mining activities are included. You may think, "well, what about HIPAA?" and this is not covered by HIPAA. HIPAA is a separate entity. HIPAA covers information from health insurance companies. And even though this information is protected, it goes back to the fact that you may have signed a permission slip and aren't aware of it.

Some of these wellness screenings require you to submit blood and other DNA containing samples. Where are these stored? Who owns the rights to these blood samples? Is your DNA becoming available for sale? Earlier we discussed the Henrietta Lacks case, and the legal status of this is unclear. What can be done with this information, and how can it be used for or against you? There is not real information on this just yet.

In 2008, the US Congress passed GIN- the Genetic Information NonDiscrimination Act of 2008. This was designed to prohibit the use of genetic information being used for health insurance or employment ("US Congress," 2008). "The Act prohibits group health plans and health insurers from denying coverage to a healthy individual or charging that person higher premiums based solely on a genetic predisposition to developing a disease in the future. The legislation also bars employers from using individuals' genetic information when making hiring, firing, job placement, or promotion decisions" ("US Congress," 2008).

Unfortunately, this is happening, whether we like it or not.
"Medical Information Bureau collects data to deny life insurance claims and life insurance policies. You can get a report for free" (MIB, n.d.) They call this an "information exchange" and claim that it's done to offer consumers and companies the best rates possible. While it is not yet proven that they are using DNA information, the operations of MIB are suspect at best. They claim that they do not use "genetic testing" information to determine whether someone is qualified for their services, yet they also state:

> MIB's members agree to share information of underwriting significance in the form of medical and avocation "codes," which are a simple form of encryption to protect the confidentiality of an individual's medical condition. Members report information to MIB using these proprietary and highly confidential codes to signify different medical conditions and other conditions (i.e., dangerous hobbies and adverse driving records) affecting the insurability of the proposed insured. These are conditions that have a significant impact on mortality (likelihood of death) or morbidity (likelihood of illness) and are reported under broad categories of medical histories or conditions. Medical records such as examination reports, attending physician statements, lab test results, x-rays, underwriting files and reasons for denial are not stored or maintained in MIB's database.

(MIB, n.d.)

Anyone can read between the lines and determine that genetic and familial history could easily (and probably are) be used to deny someone the right to an insurance claim with these types of vague statements. This is just one such company out there. They use many types of reports, including a FICO Medication Adherence score.

Today, along with a FICO credit score, FICO has now started to keep a "FICO Medication Adherence Score." How are they collecting this information? From your pharmacy. From pharmacy rewards. From your insurance companies.

"The algorithm scores patient adherence, using the prescriptions doctors write. The algorithm figures out who does or doesn't fill their prescriptions, how often patients order refills (whether we are using them too slowly or too quickly) and what those prescriptions are forward - information that indicates what diagnoses patients have had, and more.

The more adherent an individual is, the higher the score.

FICO will purchase the data used in its algorithm from large pharmacies like Express Scripts, Medco, Rite-Aid, CVS and Walgreens" (Torrey, 2016). And again, you have probably signed over your private information and given permission for this without even knowing it.

Who is going to buy Medication Adherence Scores? For starters, I would bet dollars to donuts that MIB is one of their customers. Health insurance companies are another suspect company. They can't reject any applicant for existing conditions, but they can continue to price patients out of a policy based on their health and whether they adhere to prescription taking or not. Employers could purchase the Medication Adherence Score to see how reliable you are. If you aren't taking your meds as prescribed, can you be trusted to be to work on time and be reliable? Your own doctor could even use it to dismiss you as a patient for non-adherence to treatment. (FICO, 2017)

It has been suggested that up to 50% of FICO credit reports have serious errors on them. What, then, is preventing the FICO Medication Adherence Score to not have the same problems? I can see this becoming an issue. Example: I am an identical twin. Our names are similar. Our identity numbers are one number off. Her financial information has, at times, appeared on my credit reports. Who's to say that her medical information is not also showing up on my FICO Medication Adherence Score, or other medical records? We have both had very different medical histories. This is setting up for a dangerous precedent in medical information and how it is being used. What if you have a John Doe I-V? Or George Foreman 1-IX? There is no guarantee, and I believe that more transparency is going to be required of FICO as people become more aware of these adherence scores.

One of the scariest things about the FICO Medication Adherence Score is that you are not able to opt out. In fact, I can't even locate where you can order your own score online or elsewhere.

Other ways that these types of programs could affect you? Personalized ads and ad tracking about medication adherence. Social workers showing up and determining that you are no longer fit to care for yourself (or your children, or whomever you care for) and having you placed into state custody and having your freedom and all your assets stripped away.

Another area that I hesitate to venture into is the area of children's vaccination records being sold and handed out like candy. Did you know that your children's private medical information is reported to the state, and is then sold for research data? In Michigan we have what is called the "Michigan Care Improvement Registry (MCIR)" where all information related to vaccinations is placed into a computer program, unless a parent has otherwise opted out. Information reported to this database includes, name, date of birth, height, weight, BMI, immunizations given, and who administered the immunizations. This information, minus the identifying information can then be given to research organizations and used for studies without you ever knowing about it.

On top of that, it has been determined via a FOIA request, that Pfizer has access to MCIR information.

"The Michigan Care Improvement Registry (MCIR) has the capacity to receive data for Meaningful Use Stages 1, 2 and 3 in accordance to the requirements for both 2014 and 2015 Certified Electronic Health Records Technology (CEHRT) editions" ("Meaningful Use," 2018). This means, that health care professionals that utilize MCIR can the Centers for Medicare and Medicaid offer monetary incentive programs to providers who participate in electronic medical reporting such as this. They utilize information from the public, and then report this information to government websites. (Again, sometimes without your knowledge or consent!) From the CMS website: "In 2011, the Centers for Medicare & Medicaid Services (CMS) established the Medicare and Medicaid Electronic Health Record (EHR) Incentive Programs to encourage Eligible Professionals (EPs), Eligible Hospitals, and Critical Access Hospitals (CAHs) to adopt, implement, upgrade (AIU), and demonstrate meaningful use of certified EHR technology (CEHRT)" (CMS, 2017). This, in turn, goes back to our discussion in Chapter 4 looking at how doctors are very interested in padding their pocketbooks; anything for a few extra dollars!

You can do a quick Google search to determine if your state has a program like MCIR. Most states do as electronic reporting are often mandated by state agencies.

As the quote at the beginning of this chapter says, we scream and loudly proclaim that we have medical privacy, but the reality is, is that it doesn't exist. Our bodies are for sale. Our medical records are for sale. Information about our private and most intimate details is for sale. It is up to us to make a difference. Demand change. Demand transparency. Demand medical privacy. And finally, demand a change of allowing our medical information to be available for sale.

References

Chapter 1

23AndMe. (n.d.). DNA genetic testing & analysis. Retrieved from

https://www.23andme.com/about/tos/

Askt, J. (2014, October 14). US nurse contracts Ebola. Retrieved from

https://www.the-

scientist.com/?articles.view/articleNo/41208/title/US-Nurse-

Contracts-Ebola/

Campbell Evans, Paula (October 1, 2006). Patient rights in biological

material. *BioBusiness   Legal Affairs.* Genetic Engineering News. p. 12.

Cantwell, A. (1988). AIDS and the doctors of death: An inquiry into the

origin of the AIDS   epidemic. Los Angeles: Aries Rising Press.

CDC: 2016-2017 Flu vaccine nearly 50 percent effective. (2017, February

21). Retrieved from   http://www.aafp.org/news/health-of-the-

public/20170221fluvacceffect.html

Ebola (Ebola Virus Disease). (2017, June 13). Retrieved from

https://www.cdc.gov/vhf/ebola/index.html

Emily, J. (2016, October). Nurse Nina Pham settles Ebola lawsuit against

Texas Health   Resources. Retrieved from

       https://www.dallasnews.com/news/news/2016/10/24/ebola-

nurse-nina-pham-settles-   dallas-lawsuit-claims-improper-training-

protection-invasion-privacy

GeneSight. (2017, July 11). Assurex Health's notice of privacy practices.

Retrieved from https://genesight.com/wp-

content/uploads/2017/05/notice_of_privacy_practices.pdf

Kochanek, K. D., Murphy, S. L., Xu, J., & Tejada-Vera, B. (2016). National

Vital Statistics Report. *National Vital Statistics Report, 65*(4), 1-121.

Retrieved from

       https://www.cdc.gov/nchs/data/nvsr/nvsr65/nvsr65_04.pdf.

Roan, S. (2009, April 27). Swine flu 'debacle' of 1976 is recalled. Retrieved

from   http://articles.latimes.com/2009/apr/27/science/sci-swine-

history27

Shilts, R. (1988). And the band played on: Politics, people and the AIDS

epidemic.   Harmondsworth: Penguin Books.

Skloot, R. (2010). The immortal life of Henrietta Lacks. New York:

Broadway Books.

Strauss, V. (1999, July 21). GAO to probe diversion of CDC research

funds. Retrieved from

    https://www.washingtonpost.com/archive/politics/1999/07/21

/gao-to-probe- diversion-of-cdc-research-funds/edb29fd0-3376-4218-

aacf-   949ea1a7cc18/?utm_term=.ed995392d5d8

Chapter 2

ANA Enterprise CEO Weston Announces Resignation. (2018,

    September 28). Retrieved from

    http://www.nursingworld.org/HomepageCategory/NursingInsi

    der/ANA-Enterprise-CEO-Announces-Resignation.html

American Nurses Association. (2016, March 22). American Nurses

    Association endorses Hillary Clinton for President (3/22/16).

    Retrieved from

    http://www.nursingworld.org/FunctionalMenuCategories/Med

    iaResources/PressReleases/2016-News-Releases/ANA-

    Endorses-Hillary-Clinton-for-President.html

Ernst, D. (2018, February 20). Pelosi ignores net worth inquiry after

    lecturing on 'inordinate wealth'. Retrieved from

    https://www.washingtontimes.com/news/2018/feb/20/nancy-

    pelosi-ignores-net-worth-inquiry-after-lectu/

Glassdoor. (2017). American Nurses Association reviews. Retrieved from

https://www.glassdoor.com/Reviews/American-Nurses-

Association-Reviews-E355881.htm

OpenSecrets.org. (2017). Pharmaceuticals/health products. Retrieved

from

https://www.opensecrets.org/industries/indus.php?ind=H04

Union of Concerned Scientists. (n.d.). Drug and medical device

companies have outsized influence on FDA. Retrieved from

http://www.ucsusa.org/our-work/center-science-and-

democracy/promoting-scientific-integrity/drug-companies-

influence-FDA.html#.Whxp3VNOnIV

Union Facts. (n.d.). Union Facts American Nurses Association profile,

membership, leaders, political operations, etc. Retrieved from

https://www.unionfacts.com/union/American_Nurses_Associati

on

Chapter 3

Afluria-package insert. (2014). Retrieved from

http://www.fda.gov/downloads/BiologicsBloodVaccines/Vaccin

es/ApprovedProducts/UCM263239.pdf

Brown, I. A., & Austin, D. W. (2012, September 20). Maternal transfer of

mercury to the developing embryo/fetus: Is there a safe level? Retrieved

from

http://www.tandfonline.com/doi/abs/10.1080/02772248.2012.7

24574

Bruce, D. (2016, December 21). Erie hospital to pay, rehire ex-workers

who refused flu shots.   Retrieved from

http://www.goerie.com/news/20161221/erie-hospital-to-pay-rehire-

ex-workers-who-refused-flu-shots

Centers for Disease Control. (2016, November 07). Cell-based flu

vaccines. Retrieved from

https://www.cdc.gov/flu/protect/vaccine/cell-based.htm

Centers for Disease Control. (n.d.). Health care facility HAI reporting

requirements to CMS via   NHSN-- Current or proposed

requirements. Retrieved from

https://www.cdc.gov/nhsn/PDFs/CMS/CMS-Reporting-

Requirements.pdf

Craigie, J. (2011). Competence, practical rationality and what a patient

values. *Bioethics,* 25(6), 326-333. doi:10.1111/j.1467-

8519.2009.01793.x

EEOC informal opinion letter regarding Title VII: Religious

accommodation. (2012). Retrieved from

http://www.eeoc.gov/eeoc/foia/letters/2012/religious_accomm

odation.html

Estimating seasonal influenza-associated deaths in the United States:

CDC study confirms variability of flu. (2015). Retrieved from

http://www.cdc.gov/flu/about/disease/us_flu-

related_deaths.htm#pneumonia-influenza

Food and Drug Administration. (2017, January 6). Women's health

research - List of pregnancy   exposure registries. Retrieved from

https://www.fda.gov/ScienceResearch/SpecialTopics/WomensH

ealthResearch/ucm13484   8.htm

Flu Information for Healthcare Workers. (2015). Retrieved from

https://www.dmc.org/flu-   information-for-health care-workers.html

Flu Symptoms & Complications. (2016, May 23). Retrieved from

https://www.cdc.gov/flu/about/disease/complications.htm

Fluzone. (2016, May). Retrieved from

https://www.fda.gov/downloads/biologicsbloodvaccines/vaccine

s/approvedproducts/ucm   356094.pdf

Goldman, G.S. (2013). Comparison of VAERS fetal-loss reports during three consecutive influenza seasons: Was there a synergistic fetal toxicity associated with the two-vaccine 2009/2010 season? *Human and Experimental Toxicology, 32*(5), pp. 464-475.

Grabenstein, J. D. (2013). What the world's religions teach, applied to vaccines and immune globulins. *Vaccine, 31*(16), 2011-2023. doi:http://dx.doi.org/10.1016/j.vaccine.2013.02.026

Hall, P. (2014, June 10). Lehigh County woman gets $11.6 million settlement for paralysis caused by vaccine. Retrieved from http://articles.mcall.com/2014-06-10/news/mc-lehigh-valley-vaccine-injury-settlement-20140610_1_flu-vaccine-vaccine-manufacturers-flu-shot

Hospital Inpatient Quality Reporting (IQR) Program Guide for New Facilities. (2015). Retrieved from http://www.qualityreportingcenter.com/wp-content/uploads/2015/08/IQR_Hospital-IQR-Program-Guide-for-New-Facilities_8.13.2015_Final5088.17.15.pdf

Hospital VBP program payment adjustments. (n.d.). Retrieved from http://www.medicare.gov/hospitalcompare/data/payment-adjustments.html

Influenza activity — United States, 2014–15 season and composition of the 2015–16 influenza vaccine. (2015, June 5). Retrieved from

http://www.cdc.gov/mmwr/preview/mmwrhtml/mm6421a5.htm

Interim Guidance for the Use of Masks to Control Influenza Transmission. (2009, August 1).   Retrieved from

http://www.cdc.gov/flu/professionals/infectioncontrol/maskguidance.htm

James, J. (2013). A new, evidence-based estimate of patient harms associated with hospital   care. *Journal of Patient Safety*, *9*(3), 122-128. doi:10.1097/PTS.0b013e3182948a69

Jefferson, T., Di Pietrantonj, C., Rivetti, A., Bawazeer, G., Al-Ansary, L., & Ferroni, E. (2014).

Vaccines for preventing influenza in healthy adults. *Cochrane Database Of Systematic   Reviews*, (3), doi:10.1002/14651858.CD001269.pub3

Kochanek, K., Murphy, S. L., Xu, J., & Tejada-Vera, B. (2016). Deaths: Final data for   2014. National Vital Statistics Reports, 65(4), 1-121. Retrieved from

https://www.cdc.gov/nchs/data/nvsr/nvsr65/nvsr65_04.pdf.

Landro, L. (2013). Health staffs get flu shots to avoid penalty. Retrieved

from

http://www.wsj.com/news/articles/SB10001424052702303843 1

04579169591081743318

Leading causes of death. (2015). Retrieved from

http://www.cdc.gov/nchs/fastats/leading-causes-of-death.htm

Murphy, S., Kochanek, K., Xu, J., & Heron, M. (2015, August 31). Deaths:

Final data for 2012.   Retrieved from

http://www.cdc.gov/nchs/data/nvsr/nvsr63/nvsr63_09.pdf

Murphy, S., Xu, J., & Kochanek, K. (2013, May 8). Deaths: Final data for

2010. Retrieved   from

http://www.cdc.gov/nchs/data/nvsr/nvsr61/nvsr61_04.pdf

National Institutes of Health. (1949). The Nuremberg Code. Retrieved

from

https://history.nih.gov/research/downloads/nuremberg.pdf

Niles, M., & Johnson, N. (2016). Hawthorne effect in hand hygiene

compliance   rates. *American Journal of Infection Control, 44*(6), S28-S29.

doi:10.1016/j.ajic.2016.04.190

Papple, D. (2015, October 9). Nurses' union wins battle over 'Vaccinate

Or Mask' policy: Here's why. Retrieved from

http://www.inquisitr.com/2483594/nurses-union-wins-battle-

over-vaccinate-or-mask-policy-heres-why/

Protection from flu vaccination reduced this season. (2015). Retrieved

from http://www.cdc.gov/media/releases/2015/p0115-flu-

vaccination.html

Seasonal Influenza Vaccine Effectiveness, 2005-2016. (2016, October 14).

Retrieved from

https://www.cdc.gov/flu/professionals/vaccination/effectiveness

-studies.htm

Seqirus. (2016, April). Flucelvax. Retrieved from

https://www.fda.gov/downloads/BiologicsBloodVaccines/Vacci

nes/ApprovedProducts/U   CM329134.pdf

Serres, G. D., Skowronski, D. M., Ward, B. J., Gardam, M., Lemieux, C.,

Yassi, A., . . . Carrat,   F. (2017). Influenza vaccination of health care

workers: Critical analysis of the   evidence for patient benefit

underpinning policies of enforcement. *Plos One, 12*(1).

doi:10.1371/journal.pone.0163586

The ADA: Your Employment Rights as an Individual With a Disability.
(n.d.). Retrieved from

https://www.eeoc.gov/eeoc/publications/ada18.cfm

Title VII of the Civil Rights Act of 1964. (n.d.). Retrieved from

http://www.eeoc.gov/laws/statutes/titlevii.cfm

Vaccine effectiveness - How well does the flu vaccine work? (2017).

Retrieved from

http://www.cdc.gov/flu/about/qa/vaccineeffect.htm

Vaccine injury compensation program- Frequently Asked Questions.

   (n.d.). Retrieved from

   http://www.hrsa.gov/vaccinecompensation/faq.html

World Health Organization. (2016, December 12). Influenza. Retrieved

from   http://www.who.int/biologicals/vaccines/influenza/en/

Chapter 4

American Academy of Pediatrics. (2013). Reaffirmation: Responding to

parents who refuse   immunization for their children. *Pediatrics, 131(5)*.

doi:10.1542/peds.2013-0430

Aguire, P. C. (n.d.). Understanding Capitation. Retrieved from

   https://www.acponline.org/about-acp/about-internal-

medicine/career-   paths/residency-career-

counseling/guidance/understanding-capitation

CMS. (2017, December 01). Open payments. Retrieved from

   https://www.cms.gov/openpayments/

Harris, G. (2009, September 02). Pfizer pays $2.3 billion to settle

marketing case. Retrieved   from

http://www.nytimes.com/2009/09/03/business/03health.html

Newsome, B. (2010, January 20). Dental company exploited poor children for profit, government says. Retrieved from http://gazette.com/dental-company-exploited-poor-children-for-profit-government-says/article/92717

Summers, D. (2014, January 30). Pediatrician: Vaccinate your kids-Or get out of my office. Retrieved from https://www.thedailybeast.com/pediatrician-vaccinate-your-kidsor-get-out-of-my- office

Thomas, K. (2013, November 04). J.&J. to Pay $2.2 billion in Risperdal settlement. Retrieved from http://www.nytimes.com/2013/11/05/business/johnson-johnson-to-settle- risperdal-improper-marketing-case.html

Thomas, K. (2013, December 16). Glaxo says it will stop paying doctors to promote drugs. from http://www.nytimes.com/2013/12/17/business/glaxo-says-it-will-stop-paying- doctors-to-promote-drugs.html

Chapter 5

AddictionInfo. (2010, August 29). Retrieved from https://www.addictioninfo.org/articles/507/1/Is-methadone-replacing-one-drug- addiction-with-another/Page1.html

Cost of Rehab - Paying for Addiction Treatment. (n.d.). Retrieved from

https://www.addictioncenter.com/rehab-questions/cost-of-drug-

and-alcohol-   treatment/

Gunderman, R. (2013, October 30). When physicians' careers suffer

because they refuse to   prescribe narcotics. Retrieved from

https://www.theatlantic.com/health/archive/2013/10/when-

physicians-careers-suffer-   because-they-refuse-to-prescribe-

narcotics/280995/

Ochoa, J. (2017, December 21). Their only option: Uninsured struggle to

find mental health   care. Retrieved from http://wlrn.org/post/their-

only-option-uninsured-struggle-find-   mental-health-care

Opioid Lawsuit – Government Settlements with Manufacturers & Sellers.

(n.d.). Retrieved   from https://www.levinlaw.com/government-

opioid-lawsuit

Pohl, M., & Smith, L. (2012). Chronic pain and addiction: challenging co-

occurring disorders.   *Journal Of Psychoactive Drugs, 44*(2), 119-

124.

Portenoy, R. K., & Foley, K. M. (1986). Chronic use of opioid analgesics in

non-malignant pain: Report of 38 cases. *Pain, 25*(2), 171-186.

doi:10.1016/0304-3959(86)90091-6

Chapter 6

Asbill, S., Moultry, A. M., Policastri, A., Sincak, C. A., Smith, L. S., & Ulbrich, T. R. (2016).   Debating the effectiveness and necessity of tenure in pharmacy education. *American   Journal Of Pharmaceutical Education, 80*(6), 1-6.

Bailey, M. (2016, July 20). Harvard Medical School eases rule on faculty ties to industry.   Retrieved from https://www.statnews.com/2016/05/12/harvard-med-faculty- industry-ties/

Balietti, S., Goldstone, R. L., & Helbing, D. (2016). Peer review and competition in the Art   Exhibition Game. *Proceedings of the National Academy of Sciences, 113*(30), 8414-8419. doi:10.1073/pnas.1603723113

Feilden, T. (2017, February 22). Most scientists 'can't replicate studies by their peers'.   Retrieved from http://www.bbc.com/news/science-environment-39054778

Financial Conflict of Interest Policy. (n.d.). Retrieved from   https://vpr.harvard.edu/pages/financial-conflict-interest-policy

Haug, C. J. (2015). Peer-review fraud--Hacking the scientific publication process. *New England   Journal Of Medicine, 373*(25), 2393-2395. doi:10.1056/NEJMp1512330

Herndon, N. C. (2016). Research fraud and the publish or perish world of academia. *Journal   of Marketing Channels, 23*(3), 91-96. doi:10.1080/1046669x.2016.1186469

Jacobson, R. M., Fairbrother, G., Sheldrick, R. C., & Szilagyi, P. G. (2017). The role of the peer
reviewer. *Academic Pediatrics, 17*(2), 105-106.

Kearns, C. E., Schmidt, L. A., & Glantz, S. A. (2016). Sugar industry and coronary heart disease research: A historical analysis of internal industry documents. JAMA Internal   Medicine, 176(11), 1680-1685. doi:10.1001/jamainternmed.2016.5394

Kell, J. (2016, March 29). Soda consumption falls to 30-year low in the U.S. Retrieved May 23, 2017, from http://fortune.com/2016/03/29/soda-sales-drop-11th-year/

Neimark, J. (2014, October 2). The dirty little secret of cancer research. Retrieved from http://discovermagazine.com/2014/nov/20-trial-and-error

Rong, X., & QuanQiu, W. (2016). Towards understanding brain-gut-microbiome connections   in Alzheimer's disease. *BMC Systems Biology*, 107277-285. doi:10.1186/s12918-016- 0307-y

Steen, R. (2011). Retractions in the scientific literature: Do authors deliberately commit   research fraud? *Journal of Medical Ethics, 37*(2), 113-117. Retrieved from   http://www.jstor.org/stable/23034651

Südhof, T. C. (2016). Truth in science publishing: A personal perspective. *Plos Biology, 14*(8),
1-4.

University of Pennsylvania School of Medicine. (2017, May 10). Link

between common brain disease and gut microbiome. *ScienceDaily*.

Retrieved from

www.sciencedaily.com/releases/2017/05/170510132009.htm

Wakefield, A., Murch, S., Anthony, A., Linnell, J., Casson, D., Malik, M.,

& ... Walker-Smith, J.　　　(1998). Ileal-lymphoid-nodular

hyperplasia, non-specific colitis, and pervasive

developmental disorder in children. *Lancet, 351*(9103), 637-641.

Wilson, D. (2009, March 02). Harvard medical school in ethics quandary.

Retrieved from

http://www.nytimes.com/2009/03/03/business/03medschool.ht

ml

Chapter 7

AZT's Inhuman Cost. (1989, August 27). Retrieved from

http://www.nytimes.com/1989/08/28/opinion/azt-s-inhuman-
cost.html
Bomey, N. (2016, August 25). Ex-pharma CEO Martin Shkreli defends

EpiPen price increase.　　　Retrieved from

https://www.usatoday.com/story/money/2016/08/25/martin-shkreli-

heather-bresch-mylan-epipen/89334136/

Center for Drug Evaluation and Research. (n.d.). BeSafeRx: Know your

online pharmacy - For   the media. Retrieved from

https://www.fda.gov/Drugs/ResourcesForYou/Consumers/Buy

ingUsingMedicineSaf

ely/BuyingMedicinesOvertheInternet/BeSafeRxKnowYourOnlin

ePharmacy/ucm2941   70.htm#countries

CMS. (n.d.). Costs in the coverage gap. Retrieved from

https://www.medicare.gov/part-   d/costs/coverage-gap/part-d-

coverage-gap.html

How Many Pills Do Your Elderly Patients Take Each Day? (2010,

October 04). Retrieved December 28, 2017, from

http://www.mdmag.com/conference-   coverage/aafp_2010/how-many-

pills-do-your-elderly-patients-take-each-day

Kelto, A. (2015, March 19). Why is insulin so expensive in the U.S.?

Retrieved from https://www.npr.org/sections/health-

shots/2015/03/19/393856788/why-is-u-s-   insulin-so-expensive

Tucker, M. E. (2015, March 18). Why are there no generic insulins?

Retrieved from https://www.medscape.com/viewarticle/841669

Chapter 8

CMS. (n.d.). The HCAHPS Survey – Frequently asked questions.
Retrieved from   https://www.cms.gov/medicare/quality-
initiatives-patient-assessment-

instruments/hospitalqualityinits/downloads/hospitalhcahpsfacts
heet201007.pdf

Falkenberg, K. (2016, March 24). Why rating your doctor is bad for your
health. Retrieved   from

https://www.forbes.com/sites/kaifalkenberg/2013/01/02/why-
rating-your-   doctor-is-bad-for-your-health/#794c6a4333c5

Fenton, J. J., Jerant, A. F., Bertakis, K. D., & Franks, P. (2012). The cost
of satisfaction: A   national study of patient satisfaction, health care
utilization, expenditures, and   mortality. *Archives of Internal Medicine,
172*(5), 405.   doi:10.1001/archinternmed.2011.1662

Gunderman, R. (2013, October 30). When physicians' careers suffer
because they refuse to   prescribe narcotics. Retrieved from

https://www.theatlantic.com/health/archive/2013/10/when-
physicians-careers-suffer-   because-they-refuse-to-prescribe-
narcotics/280995/

Robbins, A. (2015, April 17). The problem with satisfied patients.
Retrieved from

https://www.theatlantic.com/health/archive/2015/04/the-
problem-with-satisfied- patients/390684/

Chapter 9

CMS. (2017, November 29). Electronic Health Records (EHR) incentive programs. Retrieved   from https://www.cms.gov/Regulations-and-Guidance/Legislation/EHRIncentivePrograms/index.html

EEOC. (n.d.). EEOC's final rule on employer wellness programs and Title I of the Americans   With Disabilities Act. Retrieved January 17, 2018, from   https://www1.eeoc.gov//laws/regulations/qanda-ada-wellness-final- rule.cfm?renderforprint=1

FICO. (2017, May 23). FICO® Medication Adherence Score | FICO®. Retrieved   from http://www.fico.com/en/products/fico-medication-adherence-score

Meaningful use. (2018). Retrieved from **https://www.mcir.org/mu/**

MIB. (n.d.). The facts about MIB. Retrieved from **http://www.mib.com/facts_about_mib.html**

Torrey, T. (2016, September 7). What is the FICO Medication Adherence Score? Retrieved   from https://www.verywell.com/what-is-the-fico-medication- adherence-score-2615104

U.S. Congress. (n.d.). H.R. 493 (110th): Genetic Information Nondiscrimination Act of 2008. Retrieved from https://www.govtrack.us/congress/bills/110/hr493/summary

Appendix

<u>Appointing a Patient Advocate</u>

If you are concerned that you may not be getting the care that you were promised, or need, it may be in your best interest to appoint a patient advocate. You are probably wondering, "what is a patient advocate?" and "why would I need one?"

Simply put, a patient advocate is a person who is there to advocate for the patient. Nurses are supposed to be patient advocates, but I have seen many that do not do the job of an advocate well, or at all.

Here is a scenario for you: you are alone in the hospital, and you are confused about the treatment options being given to you. A hospital professional is pushing you (and in some cases, even threatening) to accept treatment immediately, but you want some choices and more information. Your family is lost. They are not medical professionals. No one is sure what the outcomes may be overall. Therefore, you call in your patient advocate. Your advocate, Sara Sue Smith comes in to help you. Sara is a nurse who has training in patient advocacy. She also understands many complex medical procedures and knows how to get the answers that you need. She will tell the hospital professional to back off, and help you find more information. She will also fight for you to get the treatment that you want, or help you say no if you decide to go another direction.

Here is another scenario. You are a patient in labor. The hospital staff is not following your birth plan, they are yelling at you, and they are threatening you. You are scared, in pain, nervous, and want help. You call your advocate Sara Smith. Sara shows up and tells the staff how you are going to deliver. You want to be on hands and knees, and you want to be up walking around as much as possible. Sara will let the staff know what your birth plans are and will fight for you to have the right to give birth the way that you see fit, and for the safe delivery of your baby.

Here is a sample form that you can use to download and print. You may also visit the world wide web and find similar PDF versions of this form to download and use at your discretion. I recommend having this document notarized and copies made. Have the original document placed in a safe.

<u>Appointment of Successor Patient Advocate(s)</u>

I appoint the following person(s) as my Successor Patient Advocate if my Patient
Advocate does not accept my appointment, is incapacitated, resigns or is removed.
My Successor Patient Advocate is to have the same powers and rights as my
Patient Advocate.

Full Legal Name:
Address:
Phone:
Email:

My Patient Advocate or Successor Patient Advocate may delegate his/her powers
to the next Successor Patient Advocate if he or she is not able to act.

My Patient Advocate or Successor Patient Advocate may act only if I am unable
to participate in making decisions regarding my medical, or as applicable, mental
health treatment.

Instructions for Care
1. General Instructions
My Patient Advocate shall have the authority to make all decisions and to take all
actions regarding my care, custody, medical and mental health treatment including but
not limited to the following:
a. Have access to, obtain copies of and authorize release of my medical, mental health and other personal information.
b. Employ and discharge physicians, nurses, therapists, any other health care providers, mental health professionals and other providers, and arrange to pay them reasonable compensation.

c. Consent to, refuse or withdraw for me any medical, or mental health care; diagnostic, surgical, or therapeutic procedure; or other treatment of any type or nature, including life-sustaining treatments. I understand that life-sustaining treatment includes but is not limited to breathing with the use of a machine and receiving food, water and other liquids through tubes. I also understand that these decisions could or would allow me to die.

I have listed below any specific instructions I have related to life-sustaining treatments.

Specific Instructions
My Patient Advocate is to be guided in making medical and mental health decisions for me by what I have told him/her about my personal preferences regarding my care.
Some of my preferences are recorded below and on the following pages.
a. Specific Instructions Regarding Care I DO want.

b. Specific Instructions Regarding Care I DO NOT want.

c. Specific Instructions Regarding Life-Sustaining Treatment

I understand that I do not have to choose one of the instructions
regarding life-sustaining treatment listed below. If I choose one, I will
sign below my choice. If I sign one of the choices listed below, I direct
that reasonable measures be taken to keep me comfortable and relieve
pain.

Choice 1:
I do not want my life to be prolonged by providing or continuing life-
sustaining treatment if any of the following medical conditions exist:

I am in an irreversible coma or persistent vegetative state.
I am terminally ill and life-sustaining procedures would serve only to
artificially delay my death.
Under any circumstances where my medical condition is such that the
burdens of the treatment outweigh the expected benefits.
In weighing the burdens and benefits of treatment, I want my Patient
Advocate to consider the relief of suffering and the quality of my life as
well as the extent of possibly prolonging my life.
I understand that this decision could or would allow me to die.

If this statement reflects your desires, sign here:

____

Choice 2:
I want my life to be prolonged by life-sustaining treatment unless I am in
a coma or vegetative state which my doctor reasonably believes to be
irreversible. Once my doctor has reasonably concluded that I will remain
unconscious for the rest of my life, I do not want life-sustaining treatment
to be provided or continued. I understand that this decision could or
would allow me to die.

If this statement reflects your desires, sign here:

____

Choice 3:
I want my life to be prolonged to the greatest extent possible consistent
with sound medical practice without regard to my condition, the chances I
have for recovery, or the cost of my care, and I direct life-sustaining
treatment to be provided to prolong my life.

If this statement reflects your desires, sign here:

____

d. Specific Instructions Regarding Medical Examinations

My religious beliefs prohibit a medical examination to determine whether
I am unable to participate in making medical treatment decisions. I desire
this determination to be made in the following manner:

e. Specific Instructions Regarding Anatomical Gifts
My Patient Advocate has the authority, upon or immediately before my
death,
to make an anatomical gift of all or a part of my body for transplantation
needed by another individual; for medical or dental education, research, or
the
advancement of medical or dental science; for anatomical study; or for any
other
purpose then permitted by law. This authority granted to my Patient
Advocate
shall remain following my death.

If this statement reflects your desires, sign here:

____

f. Specific Instructions Regarding Mental Health Treatment
I understand that I may, but am not required to, designate a physician
and/or
mental health practitioner to certify in writing and after examining me
that I am
unable to give informed consent to mental health treatment. If any
physician or
mental health practitioner whom I designate is unable or unwilling to
conduct
the examination and to make this determination within a reasonable time,
I
understand that the examination and determination shall be made by
another
physician or mental health practitioner, as applicable.

I prefer that the following physician(s) and/or mental health
practitioner(s)
conduct the examination (no designation is made if left blank):

____
Physician(s) and/or Mental Health Practitioner(s) Names

Regarding mental health treatment decisions, I expressly authorize my
Patient Advocate to consent to the forced administration of medication or

to inpatient hospitalization if a physician and/or mental health practitioner determine that I cannot give informed consent for the mental health care. However, I retain my right to terminate a hospitalization as a formal voluntary patient under an application executed by my Patient Advocate.

Sign your name here if you give the consent described above:

____

Patient's Signature

I understand that I may choose to waive my right to revoke my Patient Advocate designation regarding the power to make mental health treatment decisions for me only by making this waiver in this document. Even if I waive this right to revoke, I understand that by law if mental health treatment is being provided to me, it shall not continue for more than 30 consecutive days, and that this waiver does not affect my right to terminate my hospitalization as a
formal voluntary patient.

Sign here if you waive your right to revoke your Patient Advocate designation
regarding the power to make mental health treatment decisions for you:

____

Patient Signature

This document is to be treated as a Durable Power of Attorney for Health Care and
shall survive my disability or incapacity.
If I am unable to participate in making decisions for my care and there is no Patient
Advocate or Successor Patient Advocate able to act for me, I request that the
instructions I have given in this document be followed and that this document be
treated as conclusive evidence of my wishes.
It is also my intent that anyone participating in my medical or mental health
treatment shall not be liable for following the directions of my Patient Advocate that
are consistent with my instructions.
This document is signed in the state of Michigan. It is my intent that the laws of the

state of Michigan governs all questions concerning its validity, the
interpretation of its
provisions and its enforceability. I also intend that it be applied fully
possible wherever I may be.

Photocopies of this document may be relied upon as though they were
originals.

I am providing these instructions of my free will. I have not been required
to give
them to receive or have care withheld or withdrawn. I am at least
eighteen
years old and of sound mind.

Signature Date _______________________

Name: ____

Address: ____
Witness Statement and Signature

I declare that the person who signed this Designation of Patient Advocate
signed
it in my presence and is known to me. I also declare that the person who
signed
appears to be of sound mind and under no duress, fraud, or undue
influence and is
not my husband or wife, partner, child, grandchild, brother or sister. I
declare that I
am not the presumptive heir of the person who signed the previous page,
the known
beneficiary of his/her will at the time of witnessing, his/her physician or a
person
named as the Patient Advocate.

 I also declare that I am not an employee of a life or
health insurance provider for the person who signed, an employee of a
health facility
that is treating him/her, or an employee of a home for the aged where
he/she resides,
or of a community mental health services program or hospital that is
providing mental
health services to him/her, and that I am at least eighteen years old.

WITNESSES
Signature
Name
Address
Date

Signature
Name
Address
Date

Signature
Name
Address
Date

Acceptance of Patient Advocate
The Patient Advocate and Successor Patient Advocate must sign this Acceptance before
he/she may act as Patient Advocate.

I, FULL NAME HERE , agree to be the Patient Advocate for PATIENT NAME HERE
(called "Patient" in the rest of this document).
I accept the Patient's designation of me as Patient Advocate. I understand and
agree to take reasonable steps to follow the desires and instructions of the Patient as
indicated in the Designation of Patient Advocate, in other written instructions of the
Patient and as we have discussed verbally.

I also understand and agree that:

a. This designation shall not become effective unless the Patient is unable to
participate in medical or mental health treatment decisions, as applicable.
b. A Patient Advocate shall not exercise powers concerning the Patient's care,
custody, medical or mental health treatment that the Patient—if the Patient
were able to participate in the decision—could not have exercised on his or

her own behalf.

c. This designation cannot be used to make a medical treatment decision to

withhold or withdraw treatment from a Patient who is pregnant that would

result in the pregnant Patient's death.

d. A Patient Advocate may decide to withhold or withdraw treatment which would allow a Patient to die only if the Patient has expressed in a clear

and convincing manner that the Patient Advocate is authorized to make such

a decision, and that the Patient acknowledges that such a decision could or

would allow the Patient's death.

e. A Patient Advocate shall not receive compensation for the performance of his or her authority, rights, and responsibilities, but a Patient Advocate may be reimbursed for actual and necessary expenses incurred in the performance of his or her authority, rights and responsibilities.

f. A Patient Advocate shall act in accordance with the standards of care applicable to fiduciaries when acting for the Patient and shall act consistent

with the Patient's best interests. The known desires of the Patient expressed

or evidenced while the Patient can participate in medical or mental health treatment decisions are presumed to be in the Patient's best interests.

g. A Patient may revoke his or her designation at any time and in any manner

sufficient to communicate an intent to revoke.

h. A Patient may waive the right to revoke a designation as to the power to

exercise mental health treatment decisions, and if such waiver is made, the Patient's ability to revoke as to certain treatment will be delayed for 30 days

after the Patient communicates his or her intent to revoke.

i. A Patient Advocate may revoke his or her acceptance to the designation at

any time and in any manner sufficient to communicate an intent to revoke.

j. A Patient admitted to a health facility or agency has the rights enumerated in Section 20201 of the Public Health Code, 1978 PA 368, MCL 333.20201.

k. If the designation authorizes the Patient Advocate to make an anatomical

gift, the authority remains exercisable after the Patient's death. A Patient
Advocate may not exercise the authority to make an anatomical gift if the
Patient Advocate has received actual notice that the Patient expressed an
unwillingness to make the gift.
If I am unavailable to act after reasonable effort to contact me, I delegate
my
authority to the persons the Patient has designated as Successor Patient
Advocate in the
order designated. The Successor Patient Advocate is authorized to act
until I become
available to act.

PATIENT ADVOCATE
Signature
Name
Address
Home Phone
Work Phone

SUCCESSOR PATIENT ADVOCATE

Signature
Name
Address
Home Phone
Work Phone